EXPLORING THE FRONTIERS OF INNOVATION TO TACKLE MICROBIAL THREATS

PROCEEDINGS OF A WORKSHOP

Edith Amponsah, Gillian Buckley, Julie Pavlin, and Anna Nicholson, *Rapporteurs*

Forum on Microbial Threats

Board on Global Health

Health and Medicine Division

The National Academies of
SCIENCES · ENGINEERING · MEDICINE

THE NATIONAL ACADEMIES PRESS
Washington, DC
www.nap.edu

THE NATIONAL ACADEMIES PRESS 500 Fifth Street, NW Washington, DC 20001

This activity was supported by contracts between the National Academy of Sciences and Aetna Foundation, The California Endowment (#10002009), Health Resources and Services Administration (DHHS-10002817), New York State Health Foundation (#10001272), The Rippel Foundation, and Robert Wood Johnson Foundation (#10001270). Any opinions, findings, conclusions, or recommendations expressed in this publication do not necessarily reflect the views of any organization or agency that provided support for the project.

International Standard Book Number-13: 978-0-309-67533-8
International Standard Book Number-10: 0-309-67533-2
Digital Object Identifier: https://doi.org/10.17226/25746

Additional copies of this publication are available from the National Academies Press, 500 Fifth Street, NW, Keck 360, Washington, DC 20001; (800) 624-6242 or (202) 334-3313; http://www.nap.edu.

Printed in the United States of America

Suggested citation: National Academies of Sciences, Engineering, and Medicine. 2020. *Exploring the frontiers of innovation to tackle microbial threats: Proceedings of a workshop*. Washington, DC: The National Academies Press. https://doi.org/10.17226/25746.

The National Academies of

SCIENCES • ENGINEERING • MEDICINE

The **National Academy of Sciences** was established in 1863 by an Act of Congress, signed by President Lincoln, as a private, nongovernmental institution to advise the nation on issues related to science and technology. Members are elected by their peers for outstanding contributions to research. Dr. Marcia McNutt is president.

The **National Academy of Engineering** was established in 1964 under the charter of the National Academy of Sciences to bring the practices of engineering to advising the nation. Members are elected by their peers for extraordinary contributions to engineering. Dr. John L. Anderson is president.

The **National Academy of Medicine** (formerly the Institute of Medicine) was established in 1970 under the charter of the National Academy of Sciences to advise the nation on medical and health issues. Members are elected by their peers for distinguished contributions to medicine and health. Dr. Victor J. Dzau is president.

The three Academies work together as the **National Academies of Sciences, Engineering, and Medicine** to provide independent, objective analysis and advice to the nation and conduct other activities to solve complex problems and inform public policy decisions. The National Academies also encourage education and research, recognize outstanding contributions to knowledge, and increase public understanding in matters of science, engineering, and medicine.

Learn more about the National Academies of Sciences, Engineering, and Medicine at **www.nationalacademies.org**.

The National Academies of

SCIENCES · ENGINEERING · MEDICINE

PLANNING COMMITTEE ON EXPLORING THE FRONTIERS OF INNOVATION TO TACKLE MICROBIAL THREATS[1]

KENT E. KESTER (*Co-Chair*), Vice President and Head, Translational Science and Biomarkers, Sanofi Pasteur
RAFAEL OBREGÓN (*Co-Chair*), Chief of Communications for Development, United Nations Children's Fund
KEVIN ANDERSON, Senior Program Manager, Science and Technology Directorate, U.S. Department of Homeland Security
GREGORY ARMSTRONG, Director, Advanced Molecular Detection, U.S. Centers for Disease Control and Prevention
RICK BRIGHT, Director, Biomedical Advanced Research and Development Authority (BARDA), U.S. Department of Health and Human Services
JOHN BROWNSTEIN, Chief Innovation Officer and Professor, Harvard Medical School
ANDREW CLEMENTS, Deputy Director, Pandemic Influenza and Other Emerging Threats Unit, U.S. Agency for International Development
PETER DASZAK, President, EcoHealth Alliance
LORI FOSTER, Professor, Industrial-Organizational Psychology, North Carolina State University
EVA HARRIS, Professor, Division of Infectious Diseases and Vaccinology; Director, Center for Global Public Health, University of California, Berkeley
ELIZABETH D. HERMSEN, Head, Global Antimicrobial Stewardship, Merck & Co., Inc.
JAMES LAWLER, Associate Professor, Department of Internal Medicine; Director, International Programs and Innovation, University of Nebraska Medical Center College of Medicine
JONNA A. K. MAZET, Professor of Epidemiology and Disease Ecology; Executive Director, One Health Institute, School of Veterinary Medicine, University of California, Davis
THOMAS W. SCOTT, Distinguished Professor, Department of Entomology and Nematology, University of California, Davis
PAIGE E. WATERMAN, Colonel, U.S. Army, Assistant Director, Biological Threats Office of Science and Technology Policy, Executive Office of the President

---

[1] The National Academies of Sciences, Engineering, and Medicine's planning committees are solely responsible for organizing the workshop, identifying topics, and choosing speakers. The responsibility for the published Proceedings of a Workshop rests with the rapporteurs and the institution.

MARY E. WILSON, Clinical Professor of Epidemiology and Biostatistics, University of California, San Francisco, School of Medicine; Adjunct Professor, Global Health and Population, Harvard T.H. Chan School of Public Health

Health and Medicine Division Staff

GILLIAN BUCKLEY, Senior Program Officer (*from March 2020*)
EDITH AMPONSAH, Associate Program Officer
HANNAH GOODTREE, Senior Program Assistant
CECILIA MUNDACA SHAH, Project Director (*until December 2019*)
V. AYANO OGAWA, Senior Program Officer (*until December 2019*)
YAMROT NEGUSSIE, Program Officer (*until November 2019*)
STEPHEN CHUKWURAH, Senior Program Assistant (*until December 2019*)
JULIE PAVLIN, Director, Forum on Microbial Threats; Senior Director, Board on Global Health

FORUM ON MICROBIAL THREATS[1]

PETER DASZAK (*Chair*), President, EcoHealth Alliance
KENT E. KESTER (*Vice Chair*), Vice President and Head, Translational Science and Biomarkers, Sanofi Pasteur
MARY E. WILSON (*Vice Chair*), Clinical Professor of Epidemiology and Biostatistics, University of California, San Francisco, School of Medicine; Adjunct Professor, Global Health and Population, Harvard T.H. Chan School of Public Health (*until December 2019*)
KEVIN ANDERSON, Senior Program Manager, Science and Technology Directorate, U.S. Department of Homeland Security
RICK BRIGHT, Director, Biomedical Advanced Research and Development Authority (BARDA), U.S. Department of Health and Human Services
TIMOTHY BURGESS, Director, Infectious Disease Clinical Research Program, Uniformed Services University of the Health Sciences
CRISTINA CASSETTI, Deputy Division Director, Division of Microbial and Infectious Diseases, National Institute of Allergy and Infectious Diseases, National Institutes of Health
ANDREW CLEMENTS, Deputy Director, Pandemic Influenza and Other Emerging Threats Unit, U.S. Agency for International Development
MARCOS A. ESPINAL, Director, Communicable Diseases and Environmental Determinants of Health, Pan American Health Organization
KEIJI FUKUDA, School Director and Clinical Professor, The University of Hong Kong School of Public Health (*until December 2019*)
EVA HARRIS, Professor, Division of Infectious Diseases and Vaccinology; Director, Center for Global Public Health, University of California, Berkeley
ELIZABETH D. HERMSEN, Head, Global Antimicrobial Stewardship, Merck & Co., Inc.
CHANDY C. JOHN, Director, Ryan White Center for Pediatric Infectious Diseases and Global Health, Indiana University School of Medicine
RIMA F. KHABBAZ, Director, National Center for Emerging and Zoonotic Infectious Diseases, U.S. Centers for Disease Control and Prevention
MICHAEL MAIR, Acting Director, Office of Counterterrorism and Emerging Threats, U.S. Food and Drug Administration

---

[1] The National Academies of Sciences, Engineering, and Medicine's forums and roundtables do not issue, review, or approve individual documents. The responsibility for the published Proceedings of a Workshop rests with the workshop rapporteurs and the institution.

JONNA A. K. MAZET, Professor of Epidemiology and Disease Ecology; Executive Director, One Health Institute, School of Veterinary Medicine, University of California, Davis
SALLY A. MILLER, Professor of Plant Pathology and State Extension Specialist for Vegetable Pathology, Ohio Agricultural Research and Development Center, The Ohio State University
SUERIE MOON, Director of Research, Global Health Centre, Graduate Institute of International and Development Studies, Geneva
DAVID NABARRO, Advisor, Health and Sustainability, 4SD–Skills, Systems, and Synergies for Sustainable Development
RAFAEL OBREGÓN, Chief of Communications for Development, United Nations Children's Fund
KUMANAN RASANATHAN, Board Member, Health Systems Global
GARY A. ROSELLE, Chief of Medical Service, Veterans Affairs Medical Center; Director, National Infectious Disease Services, Veterans Health Administration
PETER A. SANDS, Executive Director, The Global Fund to Fight AIDS, Tuberculosis and Malaria
THOMAS W. SCOTT, Distinguished Professor, Department of Entomology and Nematology, University of California, Davis
JAY P. SIEGEL, Retired Chief Biotechnology Officer, Head of Scientific Strategy and Policy, Johnson & Johnson (*until January 2020*)
ALAN TENNENBERG, Chief Medical Officer, Johnson & Johnson Global Public Health
MATTHEW ZAHN, Medical Director, Division of Epidemiology and Assessment, Orange County Health Care Agency

National Academies of Sciences, Engineering, and Medicine Staff

GILLIAN BUCKLEY, Senior Program Officer (*from March 2020*)
EDITH AMPONSAH, Associate Program Officer
HANNAH GOODTREE, Senior Program Assistant
CECILIA MUNDACA SHAH, Project Director (*until December 2019*)
V. AYANO OGAWA, Senior Program Officer (*until December 2019*)
YAMROT NEGUSSIE, Program Officer (*until November 2019*)
STEPHEN CHUKWURAH, Senior Program Assistant (*until December 2019*)
JULIE PAVLIN, Director, Forum on Microbial Threats; Senior Director, Board on Global Health

Reviewers

This Proceedings of a Workshop was reviewed in draft form by individuals chosen for their diverse perspectives and technical expertise. The purpose of this independent review is to provide candid and critical comments that will assist the National Academies of Sciences, Engineering, and Medicine in making each published proceedings as sound as possible and to ensure that it meets the institutional standards for quality, objectivity, evidence, and responsiveness to the charge. The review comments and draft manuscript remain confidential to protect the integrity of the process.

We thank the following individuals for their review of this proceedings:

CHANDY C. JOHN, Indiana University School of Medicine
RIMA F. KHABBAZ, U.S. Centers for Disease Control and Prevention

Although the reviewers listed above provided many constructive comments and suggestions, they were not asked to endorse the content of the proceedings nor did they see the final draft before its release. The review of this proceedings was overseen by **DAVID R. CHALLONER,** University of Florida. He was responsible for making certain that an independent examination of this proceedings was carried out in accordance with standards of the National Academies and that all review comments were carefully considered. Responsibility for the final content rests entirely with the rapporteurs and the National Academies.

Acknowledgments

The workshop summarized in this proceedings is the product of many valuable contributions. Special thanks go to the presenters and discussants who gave generously of their time and expertise to make the event possible. A full list of the speakers and moderators and their biographical information may be found in Appendix C.

Contents

Boxes and Figures

BOXES

FIGURES

Acronyms and Abbreviations

AFP	acute flaccid paralysis
AI	artificial intelligence
AMP Health	Aspen Management Partnership for Health
AMR	antimicrobial resistance
BARDA	Biomedical Advanced Research and Development Authority
CDC	U.S. Centers for Disease Control and Prevention
CDDEP	Center for Disease Dynamics, Economics & Policy
CEPI	Coalition for Epidemic Preparedness Innovations
CHRF	Child Health Research Foundation
cVDPV	circulating vaccine-derived polio virus
DARPA	Defense Advanced Research Projects Agency
DoD	U.S. Department of Defense
DRC	Democratic Republic of the Congo
EHP	Ebola Host Project
ESKAPE pathogens	*Enterococcus faecium, Staphylococcus aureus, Klebsiella pneumoniae, Acinetobacter baumannii, Pseudomonas aeruginosa,* and *Enterobacter species* pathogens
ETU	Ebola treatment unit

FDA	U.S. Food and Drug Administration
FIND	Foundation for Innovative New Diagnostics
HBV	hepatitis B virus
HCV	hepatitis C virus
HIV	human immunodeficiency virus
HPV	human papillomavirus
IPV	inactivated polio vaccine
JJDC	Johnson & Johnson Development Corporation
JPEO-CBRND	Joint Program Executive Office for Chemical, Biological, Radiological and Nuclear Defense
LMIC	low- and middle-income country
MERS	Middle East respiratory syndrome
NAP-AMR	national action plan for antimicrobial resistance
NGO	nongovernmental organization
NGS	next-generation sequencing
OPV	oral polio vaccine
PCR	polymerase chain reaction
PHEIC	public health emergency of international concern
qPCR	quantitative polymerase chain reaction
SPARK	Shared Platform for Antibiotic Research and Knowledge
USAID	U.S. Agency for International Development
VAPP	vaccine-associated paralytic polio
VDPV	vaccine-derived polio virus
WHO	World Health Organization

1

Introduction

Over the past century, advances in science and technology have helped reduce the threat from infectious diseases. Advances in genomics, robotics, imaging, geographical information systems, and other areas have changed development of diagnostics, vaccines, and therapeutics. They have also changed processes such as those for health surveillance interventions to prevent, treat, and control infectious diseases. These innovations range from small, community-based pilot projects to large-scale applications of advanced technologies using cutting-edge data analytics. Specific examples include use of mobile health applications to improve service delivery on the ground and to navigate the continuum of care (see Chapter 4); predictive modeling to inform infectious disease surveillance and outbreak response; and the use of unbiased metagenomics sequencing to counter microbial threats (see Chapter 3). Despite these advances, infectious diseases continue to cause significant morbidity and mortality worldwide. Some important questions must be answered to make the most of the innovations of the past decades. Many lifesaving innovations are not reaching those who need them (Roscigno et al., 2012). Even when they do, change can be slow to take hold because of social and cultural barriers, weak health care and data infrastructure, poor communication, limited regulatory and enforcement capacity, and other problems. Wide and lasting uptake of any intervention depends on community engagement (Roscigno et al., 2012).

There is also a problem of incentives for innovation. Some interventions, such as medical product development, have obvious appeal to industry and academia, but many do not. Changes in incentive structure for neglected areas may be needed. For example, in the United States reimbursement for diagnostics is calculated in reference to the cost to the laboratory of running the test, not the end value of the diagnostic information gained (Dzau et al., 2016). Changes to incentive structures could spur innovation and combat infectious disease.

People today live in a time of unprecedented global connection. The extent and reach of global communications, travel, manufacturing, and distribution systems have improved quality of life around the world. They also allow microbial threats to escalate at a speed that far outpaces the ability of scientists' or policy makers' countermeasures. The recent coronavirus pandemic has made this point abundantly clear. As diverse stakeholders from different sectors and disciplines continue to discover, develop, deliver, and adopt innovations to counter microbial threats, collaboration and sharing of best practices are important to push the field forward. More specifically, a One Health[1] approach is important for the successful implementation, uptake, and impact of advancements to combat microbial threats.

WORKSHOP OBJECTIVES

On December 4–5, 2019, a planning committee under the auspices of the Forum on Microbial Threats at the National Academies of Sciences, Engineering, and Medicine held a 1.5-day public workshop titled Exploring the Frontiers of Innovation to Tackle Microbial Threats.[2] The workshop examined major advances in scientific, technological, and social innovations against microbial threats. Such innovations include diagnostics, vaccines (both development and production), and antimicrobials, as well as nonpharmaceutical interventions and changes in surveillance. Workshop speakers and discussants drew from government, academic, private, and nonprofit backgrounds. Specifically, this workshop featured invited presentations and discussions on the following topics:[3]

---

[1] One Health is a collaborative, multisectoral, and transdisciplinary approach with the goal of achieving optimal health outcomes. One Health requires collaboration at the local, regional, national, and global levels and the recognition of the interconnection between people, plants, and their shared environments (CDC, 2020).

[2] The planning committee's role was limited to planning the workshop, and the Proceedings of a Workshop was prepared by the workshop rapporteurs as a factual summary of what occurred at the workshop. Statements, recommendations, and opinions expressed are those of individual presenters and participants, and are not necessarily endorsed or verified by the National Academies of Sciences, Engineering, and Medicine, and they should not be construed as reflecting any group consensus.

[3] The full Statement of Task is available in Appendix A.

- Detection and diagnostic tools that empower early treatment and other beneficial steps;
- Methods and tools such as predictive modeling, digital platforms, and precision public health, and how they might be best used;
- Methods that account for social and behavioral factors related to microbial threats;
- Communication and structural strategies to improve access to and use of behavior change for preparedness and response;
- Data and modeling insights for practitioners in diverse settings, particularly at the community level;
- Models and indicators that measure the extent to which innovations are successful; and
- Ways to stimulate meaningful collaboration and communication among multilateral organizations, national governments, the private sector, and civil society.

ORGANIZATION OF THE PROCEEDINGS OF THE WORKSHOP

In accordance with National Academies policy, the workshop participants did not venture conclusions or recommend actions, focusing instead on lively discussion. This report summarizes said discussion. Specifically, Chapter 2 presents the workshop's two keynote addresses, using examples of polio and Ebola virus disease to illustrate how sharp changes can alter the course of an outbreak. Chapter 3 features case studies on global vector control, predictive modeling, metagenomics sequencing, and mobile health diagnostic tools. Chapter 4 examines barriers to timely data sharing and ways to facilitate behavior change among health workers and patients and in communities. Chapter 5 explores strategies for spurring innovation in surveillance systems, antibiotic discovery, and diagnostic tests, as well as regulatory tools to tackle antimicrobial resistance. Chapters 6 and 7 focus on translating innovative ideas to action, with Chapter 6 giving highlights from the panel on barriers to innovation and new forms of partnership and Chapter 7 summarizing the panel on accelerating research and development. Chapter 8 provides visionary statements on priorities for innovation.

2

Pivotal Role of Innovations in Tackling Microbial Threats: Lessons from Past Outbreaks

The workshop opened with two keynote addresses from speakers who explored how innovations can be pivotal in changing the course of an outbreak. Ananda Bandyopadhyay, program officer, Bill & Melinda Gates Foundation, described lessons learned from innovations in polio eradication over the past several decades. Jonathan Towner, team lead, disease ecology group, viral special pathogens branch, U.S. Centers for Disease Control and Prevention (CDC), examined the role of innovation on the ground in the fight against the Ebola virus, with a focus on the outbreak in West Africa (2014–2016) and the outbreak in eastern Democratic Republic of the Congo (DRC) that began in 2018.

LESSONS LEARNED FROM INNOVATION IN POLIO ERADICATION

Ananda Bandyopadhyay explored lessons learned from the global effort to achieve polio eradication over the past several decades, with a focus on how innovation can be leveraged in practical, impactful ways. He explained that disease eradication can be defined in different ways, but a simple approach is to define it as a permanent reduction of the worldwide incidence of a given infection to zero (Cochi and Dowdle, 2013). Until and unless the three criteria of zero incidence, permanency, and global scale are satisfied, a disease cannot be categorized as eradicated, he continued. Bandyopadhyay noted that the only human disease that has been eradicated is smallpox (Cochi and Dowdle, 2013). In contrast, polio is an acute viral illness that is passed from person to person, primarily through contact with feces; is highly subclinical; and although very infectious, it presents with the characteristic signs and symptoms of paralysis in only a small subset of those infected—about 1 in 200 infections (WHO, 2019a). He warned that as long as polio exists somewhere in the world, it is just a plane ride away from the countries or regions that have eliminated polio. As Bandyopadhyay explained, immunization is the only way to prevent the disease, and there is no cure for the disease, while rehabilitative therapy is the only treatment option for people who have already been paralyzed with polio (WHO, 2019a).

Progress in the Eradication of Polio

Bandyopadhyay provided an overview of the substantial progress to date toward the eradication of polio worldwide. A cadre of 20 million volunteers deliver vaccinations that reach around 400 million children each year, resulting in the prevention of paralysis on a large scale of about 18 million people who would have been paralyzed had they not been vaccinated (DFID, 2019). Wild polio cases have declined by 99.9 percent over the past 30 years, from 350,000 cases across 125 countries in 1988 to 33 cases reported in 2018 (WHO, 2019a). When the eradication program started in 1988 with the formation of the Global Polio Eradication Initiative, roughly 1,000 cases of paralysis related to polio were being reported every day, he noted. He attributed the remarkable scale of decrease in the number of paralysis cases to the eradication program, but noted that the effort has yet to achieve eradication, and there is still work to be done.

A challenge in addressing polio is that it is a combination of many diseases from the surveillance, diagnostic, and prevention perspectives, said Bandyopadhyay. Polio has been broadly categorized into the wild or naturally occurring disease type, which is further subcategorized into wild poliovirus types 1, 2, and 3. Wild types 2 and 3 were certified as eradicated in 2015 and 2019, respectively (WHO, 2019a,b). However, wild polio type 1 is still actively circulating, has the highest case-infection ratio, and spreads rapidly (WHO, 2019b). He explained that an additional burden of polio disease is related to the oral polio vaccine (OPV), referred to as OPV-related polio, which is subclassified into two categories. Vaccine-associated paralytic polio myelitis (VAPP) is an aberrant neuroparalytic reaction to the oral live polio vaccine virus in an individual who received the vaccine or was in close contact with the vaccine (WHO, 2019c). The overall risk of VAPP in low- and middle-income countries is about 1 case per 4–5 million OPV doses (Platt et al., 2014). The other subcategory, vaccine-derived polio viruses (VDPVs), are revertant strains of the live OPV virus that are transmitted from one person to another, particularly in settings of very low population immunity (WHO, 2019c). Through serial transmission, the viruses become revertant and neurovirulent. Most VDPVs are circulating (cVDPVs), with type 2 cVDPVs accounting for about 90 percent of all cVDPVs (WHO, 2019c). He explained that cVDPVs are essential public health threats because they revert and become transmissible from person to person and can also cause paralysis.

The endgame phase of polio eradication requires taking into account these different subcategories of polio, Bandyopadhyay said. Although VAPP and VDPVs are public health threats of major concern, they are rare, so the OPV is still the mainstay of interrupting person-to-person transmission in high-risk settings. However, in populations with sustained low levels of population immunity, OPV strains can lead to paralysis or transmission. A balance needs to be struck between these two considerations, he said.[1]

Innovations in Polio Surveillance, Diagnostics, and Strategic Approaches

Bandyopadhyay explained that because polio is a highly subclinical disease, surveillance is critical. He explained that the overall purpose of polio surveillance is to detect in a timely manner any circulation of polio viruses in any part of the world. The Bill & Melinda Gates Foundation polio program closely tracks the polio virus in around 70 countries by testing paralyzed children and collecting environmental samples to detect virus transmission, he explained. Two forms of polio surveillance are typically used. Acute flaccid paralysis (AFP) surveillance is a clinical syndromic surveillance system whereby reports of sudden-onset paralysis in a specified age group are investigated. Environmental surveillance involves collecting sewage samples from strategically selected areas in different countries to rule out or confirm the existence of polio viruses (Bill & Melinda Gates Foundation, n.d.). He added that multiple countries contribute to polio surveillance formally or informally, with support from an extensive global network of around 150 accredited laboratories. Another objective of polio surveillance is to generate evidence to support the certification process of eradication. Maintaining an adequate quality of surveillance through appropriate methods can help identify prolonged periods without detection and contribute to the documentation around certification of polio-free status.

Many innovations are ongoing or under development in the spectrum of polio surveillance, said Bandyopadhyay. Methods to improve electronic and mobile phone–based reporting systems include the SMS-based Auto-Visual AFP Detection and Reporting project, Integrated Supportive Supervision, and the eSURV electronic surveillance tool. New tools have also been developed for sewage collection and filtration. Innovations in data and analytics include site characterization and sensitivity assessment as well as digital tools, such as digital elevation model databases, geospatial applications, and

[1] This was updated after prepublication release to remove a figure.

facial recognition technology. New direct detection and molecular methods include next-generation sequencing, MinION platforms, and methodologies that would enhance the environmental surveillance technologies. He said that these innovations are facilitating earlier and more sensitive detection, as well as creating integrated methods of detection in which polio surveillance can be combined with surveillance systems like antimicrobial resistance or typhoid surveillance.

Bandyopadhyay emphasized that despite these exciting innovations, real-world polio surveillance on the ground is largely done using traditional methods that require workers to seek out and manually transport patients to care, often across difficult terrain. He explained that to reach and protect more children, the polio program is implementing innovative strategies to achieve the aim of vaccinating every child. For instance, teams are deployed house to house as well as to transit points and health centers to vaccinate children. In areas that are high risk, the programs engage community mobilizers and religious leaders to help ensure that communities will accept the vaccine.

Innovations in Vaccines for Polio Prevention

Bandyopadhyay provided an overview of the spectrum of current innovations in vaccines, prevention, and immunologic interventions (Bandyopadhyay et al., 2015). Research on inactivated polio vaccines (IPVs) is looking to reduce costs, to increase supply, to make the vaccines more immunogenic, and to improve the delivery technologies. Clinical studies are being planned or are under way to evaluate aluminum salts and other adjuvants for IPV, to find novel routes of IPV administration that can be used concomitantly with other vaccines (e.g., disposable jet injectors and microneedle patches), and to create IPV from less infectious or noninfectious sources, such as Sabin and virus-like particles. Antiviral therapies are being developed for people who are immunodeficient and for chronic excretors who shed polio virus for long periods. He explained that antiviral therapies hold promise in interrupting the shedding and reducing the risk of community spread.

A novel genetically stabilized OPV is currently in development to strengthen outbreak control by reducing the risk of VDPVs and VAPP, said Bandyopadhyay. These vaccines are developed with inherent qualities of genetic stability, so they are more stable than the Sabin OPVs and have a lower risk of reverting into neurovirulence. He noted that this is the first new OPV development effort in about 60 years since the licensure of the Sabin vaccine. Human clinical trials began in 2017 and target-population data were generated in 2019. This effort is a large-scale partnership across many organizations and has enabled accelerated development of this vaccine to counter the threat of VDPVs. A first-in-human study was recently conducted in Belgium, where 30 individuals stayed for approximately 30 days in contained settings with extensive monitoring to understand the characteristics of the new vaccine virus strains (Van Damme et al., 2019a). Preliminary results are all promising, he said (Van Damme et al., 2019b). Researchers found clear evidence of replication in the gut and of immunogenicity. The vaccine is more genetically stable and less neurovirulent compared with the Sabin OPV, which were primary aims of developing the new vaccine.

Looking Forward to Eradicating Polio

Bandyopadhyay remarked that although multiple vaccine options are now a reality—OPV, IPV, and potentially the novel oral polio vaccine—this will not necessarily solve the issue of eradication because the core issue is vaccination, not vaccines. Regardless of a vaccine's quality, it is not effective while contained in a vial. The difference is made by people who hand carry the vaccines to children, often through seemingly impassible conditions. He lauded these people working on the ground as the champions and sources of real-world, practical innovations that have contributed to the dramatic reduction in polio cases worldwide. Despite the historic progress in reducing polio transmission, Bandyopadhyay remarked that overcoming the remaining challenges to achieve and sustain eradication will depend on concerted global efforts as well as innovation around new surveillance methodologies, vaccine formulations, and delivery technologies. The risk of reintroduction and resurgence of eradicated types of polio will also need to be managed carefully. Finally, he emphasized that the development and deployment of new tools and technologies will need to be tailored based on local need and feasibility in underserved areas—innovative strategies have to be rooted in the ground if they are to reach the last child.

ADVANCING INNOVATION ON THE GROUND IN THE FIGHT AGAINST EBOLA

In his keynote address, Jonathan Towner focused on the role of innovation on the ground in the fight against the Ebola virus. He explained that Ebola virus disease is a severe, often fatal disease with initial symptoms that are nonspecific: fever, severe headache, fatigue, muscle pain, vomiting, diarrhea, and abdominal pain. Unexplained hemorrhage is one of the disease's main features, but it only occurs in less than half of cases, he clarified. The incubation period of the disease ranges between 2 and 21 days with an average of 8 to 10 days (CDC, 2019a). The Ebola virus is transmitted primarily via direct contact through broken skin or unprotected mucous membranes with blood or body fluids, including but not limited to urine, saliva, sweat, feces, vomit, semen, and breast milk (CDC, 2019a). It can also be spread through contaminated objects, such as needles and syringes, as well as through infected animals, including apes, monkeys, and possibly bats (CDC, 2019a). Follow-up studies of survivors of the 2014 outbreak in West Africa show that the virus can persist in semen for long periods after recovery (Crozier, 2016). Historically, case fatality rates from Ebola range from to 25 to 90 percent (WHO, 2020).

Origin and Ecology of Ebola Virus

Towner explained that there are six different species of Ebola virus in the genus *Ebolavirus* within the family of filoviruses. The *Zaire ebolavirus* was the cause of the outbreak in West Africa, but three other species are known to have caused human disease: *Sudan ebolavirus*, *Tai Forest ebolavirus*, and *Bundibugyo ebolavirus*. The *Reston ebolavirus* and the *Bombali ebolavirus* are not known to cause disease in humans at this point, he said. The first filovirus, discovered in 1967, was the *Marburgvirus* species, which causes high-fatality disease like the *Zaire ebolavirus* and has been responsible for several relatively large outbreaks. The origin of the Ebola virus remains poorly understood, he added. Various spillover events have been linked to contact with infected nonhuman primates, but the original source is thought to be the bat, which is supported by the discovery of the *Bombali ebolavirus* in Sierra Leone, Guinea, and Kenya. Further support comes from findings that the Egyptian fruit bat (Egyptian rousette) is the natural reservoir for at least 25 different *Marburgvirus* isolates (Amman et al., 2012; Swanepoel et al., 2007; Towner et al., 2009).

Epidemiology of Ebola Virus Outbreaks

Towner said that the majority of filovirus outbreaks have occurred in the equatorial region of Central Africa, including the 2014 outbreak in West Africa at the nexus of Guinea, Liberia, and Sierra Leone. The first documented outbreak of Ebola virus occurred in 1976 and regular outbreaks have occurred since, including an ongoing outbreak in the eastern part of DRC that is the second largest ever recorded (CDC, 2019b). He explained that the current outbreak in DRC began in July 2018 and was ongoing as of December 2019, meaning that it has persisted much longer than typical outbreaks, which tended to last no longer than 3 months. The epidemic curve of the DRC outbreak also differs from the 2014 outbreak in West Africa; although the latter was also lengthy in comparison to previous outbreaks, it was also more explosive than the DRC outbreak in terms of the number of cases (see Figure 2-1). As a result, the West Africa outbreak tested the public

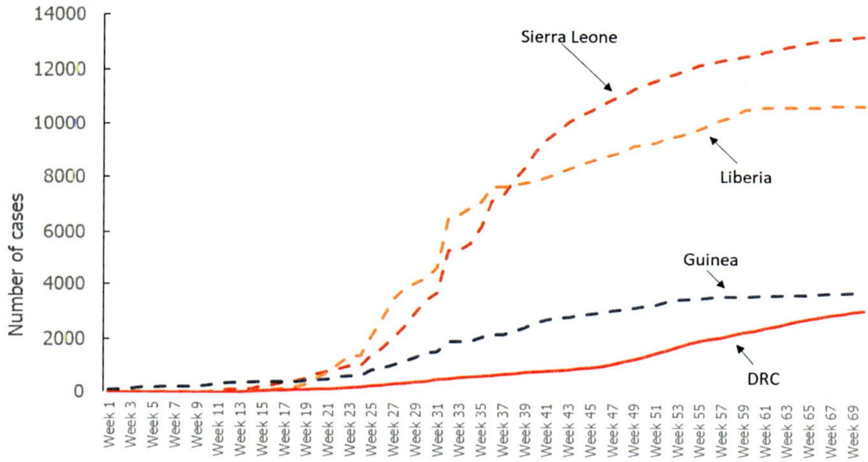

FIGURE 2-1 Epidemic curve of Ebola virus disease in the West Africa outbreak (2014–2016) and the Democratic Republic of the Congo (2018–present).
NOTE: DRC = Democratic Republic of the Congo.
SOURCES: Towner presentation, December 4, 2019; data from the U.S. Centers for Disease Control and Prevention Viral Special Pathogens Branch Emergency Operation Center for Ebola Epidemic Team.

health infrastructure of the affected countries and led the United States and Europe's exportation of multiple clinicians and health care workers for the first time. He noted that 900 of the total 28,000 cases during that outbreak were health care workers.

Progress in Diagnostics, Genomics, and Case Investigations for Ebola Virus

Towner outlined progress in diagnostics, genomics, and case investigations for Ebola virus disease. The classic response to Ebola focuses on stopping human-to-human transmission and isolating infected patients, as well as contact tracing and patient management. Aggressive infection control practices in homes and health care settings, safe burial practices, community engagement, and good data management are also major components of Ebola outbreak control. He explained that the mobile laboratory emerged as the hub for polymerase chain reaction (PCR) diagnostics during the outbreak in Gulu, Uganda, in 2000. Until the West Africa outbreak, the Gulu outbreak of 425 cases had been the largest on record. CDC fielded a team to St. Mary's Lacor Hospital in Gulu and established a laboratory that consisted of the antigen capture and ELISA[2] methods (immunoglobulin G and immunoglobulin M), he continued. These methods had been used before, but they had never been done in PCR for acute-case diagnostics that were focused on finding infected people as quickly as possible. This was done singly in phenol extractions, nested PCR gel boxes, and some marine gels, which are now antiquated technologies.

Not long after that outbreak ended in 2001, there was a major push to develop higher-throughput platforms for detecting potential bioterrorism agents, with Ebola, Marburg, and filoviruses as high priorities. This drove the development of high-throughput RNA extraction and Ebola detection through the titration of Ebola Zaire in whole blood over a 6-log range, which were later used during the Marburg virus outbreak in Angola in 2005—the first time these high-throughput platforms were used in the field. He noted that this response also included the first widespread use of oral swabs for detecting Ebola or filovirus patients, albeit with some controversy.

Towner explained that the 2014 West Africa Ebola virus outbreak spurred an all-hands-on-deck approach to field diagnostics, with laboratories from different countries fielding different PCR methodologies. CDC helped provide some of the high-throughput testing capability to a South African laboratory at Lakka in Freetown, Sierra Leone. CDC also fielded a "hot" laboratory in Bo, Sierra Leone, that was very spartan but highly effective. The Bo laboratory converted a small house into a laboratory with 96-well MagMAX traction platforms and a Biorad 96 real-time PCR machine, which was resistant to the brownouts that occurred frequently.

Ultimately, the Bo laboratory remained operational for more than 400 days, supported by 28 teams of personnel from 17 different branches throughout CDC. They processed more than 27,000 specimens over that period, sometimes processing 150–200 samples per day. He noted that a limiting step was assessing the data from case investigation forms and trying to read illegible handwriting, which monopolized time that could have been spent on diagnostic testing. The diagnostic testing included more than 500 semen specimens to assess the viral persistence in male survivors as well as samples from the Ebola vaccine trials that were ongoing at the time.

Field Diagnostic Laboratory Challenges in the West Africa Outbreak

Towner described some of the challenges they encountered while running the field diagnostic laboratory. Some issues related to the types of specimens and sample transport, which had to be managed in impromptu and ad hoc ways—from motorbikes to helicopters—in the face of the large

[2] The enzyme-linked immunosorbent assay (ELISA) is a commonly used immunological assay used to measure antigens, proteins, and antibodies in biological samples.

and dynamic West Africa outbreak. There were additional challenges related to the assays. Many different real-time PCR assays were being used across multiple laboratory networks, which necessitated attempts to standardize not only assays but also quality-control proficiency panels to identify poor performers. CDC distributed panels in Sierra Leone and Guinea and found that two of the six laboratories in Sierra Leone had 10 percent incorrect results, which enabled them to implement improvements.

Different assays also had implications for different cutoffs and interpretations in terms of criteria for releasing patients from overcrowded Ebola treatment units (ETUs). He said that health care workers were forced to make difficult decisions in certain circumstances: for example, setting criteria for release that a patient had to be clinically well and PCR negative *or* have a cycle threshold value of less than 35 if the ETU was at capacity and beds were at a premium. To create some correlation and decrease the risk of false positives and false negatives, ETUs developed a two-target Ebola assay and used cell RNA (β 2M or RNaseP) PCR controls. He noted that this turned out to be useful in the deployment of Ebola glycoprotein expressing vaccines by providing the capacity to differentiate between vaccinated and truly infected individuals.

Use of GeneXpert in the Democratic Republic of the Congo Outbreak

GeneXpert (Cepheid) is a cartridge-based platform that has now been implemented widely in the current outbreak in eastern DRC and seems to be working well, said Towner (Pettitt et al., 2017; Raftery et al., 2018; Semper et al., 2016; van Vuren et al., 2016). It is a very sensitive real-time assay with a turnaround time of 98 minutes; it accepts whole-blood or buccal swab specimens. The cartridge component makes disposal and management of the sample and remnants more manageable than other platforms. More than 120,000 field tests had been performed in DRC as of November 2019, said Towner. A caveat with GeneXpert, Towner continued, is that the only commercially available filovirus assay is for Ebola Zaire, but suggested that assays for other filoviruses will be developed.

Using Next-Generation Sequencing to Fight Ebola

Towner remarked that virus whole-genome sequencing is now possible in the field with rapid turnaround time. This next-generation sequencing (NGS) was a valuable innovation in fighting Ebola in West Africa in the later stages of the outbreak when researchers were dealing with unexplained clusters that emerged separately from any known ongoing transmission (Diallo et al., 2016; Goldstein et al., 2018; Towner et al., 2008). For example, molecular field epidemiology conducted using MinION, a handheld NGS platform, enabled researchers to have full-length genomes within 24 hours to investigate an unexplained cluster in Guinea. This genetic fingerprint of the virus was used to determine that it was a case of sexual transmission originating from a male survivor who was still shedding infectious virus 500 days after convalescence. Towner explained that this technology saves resources by narrowing down epidemiological investigations and establishing whether a virus is newly introduced, a spillover, or part of a previously unknown lengthy chain of transmission.

NGS has also been used effectively in pathogen discovery, for both the *Bundibugyo ebolavirus* in 2007 in Uganda and the *Bombali ebolavirus* in 2017 in Sierra Leone. NGS enables rapid whole-genome genetic characterization that can assess how well current diagnostic assays will be able to perform against a newly emergent virus. Knowledge of the full-length genome can also be used to rescue and test viruses when clinical samples are not available, or if samples are available but people are reluctant to handle or transport them, he said. To test truant antivirals or evaluate how well the current diagnostic assays work, the virus can be rescued from an infectious clone. A recent study tested diagnostic assays with a known mutation in a circulating virus as well as testing potential therapeutic monoclonal antibodies (McMullan et al., 2019).

Innovation in Case Detection

Simple innovations can also be highly effective, said Towner. For instance, a mobile case investigation app—the Ebola Exposure Window Calculator—has been developed to support epidemiologists by estimating the period of time during which a person could have been exposed to the Ebola virus. The information provided by this tool can be used in collaboration with other known information about a person to identify potential cases of infection.

Innovation in Capacity Building and Infection Control

Towner emphasized that investing long term in foreign diagnostic laboratory infrastructure can dramatically reduce the size, duration, and cost of outbreaks of emerging infectious diseases. Since 2010, CDC has invested in the Uganda Virus Research Institute to establish and maintain an enhanced comprehensive surveillance and diagnostics program for viral hemorrhagic fevers (CDC, 2019c). The investment has had a substantial effect by diminishing the scope of outbreaks, decreasing the number of cases, and reducing the time it takes to identify the agent of an outbreak. Towner noted that more than 1,000 health care workers have been infected with Ebola virus during the West Africa and DRC outbreaks. To improve infection control and protect health care workers, CDC and other agencies developed a training course for workers going into the field (Narra et al., 2017). The course consists of a didactic component as well as practical, hands-on training conducted in full protective equipment to simulate activities such as patient care, waste disposal, and disinfection.

Innovation in Vaccines and Therapeutics

Innovations in Ebola vaccines and therapeutics are under way and appear to be effective, said Towner. It was first demonstrated in 2000 that Ebola virus disease could be prevented by a vaccine (Sullivan et al., 2000). A new vaccine—a live attenuated recombinant vesicular stomatitis virus—is now being implemented in eastern DRC, with more than 250,000 doses already administered. Initial reports suggest that its efficacy is greater than 97 percent. Towner surmised that because the vaccine was rolled out early on in the DRC outbreak, it may have had a dramatic effect in attenuating the trajectory of the virus compared to the West Africa outbreak.

Another simple but effective innovation was developed in response to the Gates Millennium Challenge—a portable cooler that can keep the vaccine at the necessary temperature of –60 degrees Celsius for 7 days in tropical temperatures, even with repeated entries into the unit (Jusu et al., 2018). This was valuable during vaccine efforts, he said. Towner concluded with optimism that Zaire Ebola may soon be treatable. Two antibody-based cocktails hold promise as therapeutics for Zaire Ebola virus disease, said Towner. Ridgeback Biotherapeutics's mAb114 and Regeneron Pharmaceuticals's REGN-EB3 appear to decrease mortality rates by half compared to rates without those treatments (Kupferschmidt, 2019).

DISCUSSION

Peter Daszak, president of EcoHealth Alliance, noted that the current Ebola outbreak in DRC is larger and longer lasting than any previous outbreak in the region. He asked about the likelihood of future outbreaks being long-term, chronic threats or explosive outbreaks that are more similar to the 2014 outbreak in West Africa. Towner replied that one of those issues, the likelihood of spillover, has more to do with interaction with the reservoir. In the West Africa outbreak, the explosion occurred when the virus entered into the major population centers and overwhelmed the system's ability to respond in a timely way to control the outbreak through contact tracing, isolation, and other activities. It also required the international community to deal with the challenges involved in engaging with three different governments simultaneously.

He suggested that the current outbreak in eastern DRC could have been quelled in 2018 if contact tracing had been conducted effectively, but it was not possible owing to the insecure environment. Dozens of militia groups operate in the area and at least two ETUs were burned down and attacked, leading many of the international teams to pull out of the area. Cases who are not found cannot be isolated, protracting the outbreak even though the new vaccine is available. He added that fortunately, the population centers in DRC are not as large as Conakry, Freetown, and Monrovia.

Jyoti Joshi, head of the South Asia Center for Disease Dynamics, Economics & Policy, commented on the differences between the two diseases: polio being a slow and persistent threat, while Ebola was a sudden and huge threat. The innovation in the response to Ebola tended to involve laboratories reaching out to people rather than vice versa. Both cases demonstrate that innovations need to synergize with local context or reach will be limited. Joshi asked about how to implement innovations in a context-appropriate way. Bandyopadhyay remarked that each context is different, and each approach should be evaluated and adapted as it is implemented. This involves understanding the geopolitical context, engaging local communities, and ensuring local ownership of programs.

He said that the current concerted, integrated drive toward immunization has benefited the polio program, particularly in endemic areas. In terms of diagnostics, he suggested relying on culture-based methods because they are highly specific and sensitive for diseases such as polio, in which a single case can trigger an outbreak. However, as the number of polio cases continues to decrease, interest is growing in direct detection. Pilots are already under way to explore this molecular method of detection and to bring the laboratory closer to the field, but the advantages of these innovations need to be balanced with the need for specificity and sensitivity in planning for outbreak response.

James Lawler, director, International Programs and Innovation, Global Center for Health Security, University of Nebraska, highlighted the cross-cutting issue of misinformation campaigns that contributed to the outbreak of polio in northern Nigeria, hindered Ebola outbreak control efforts in eastern DRC, and is currently driving measles outbreaks in Europe and the United States. Towner commented that community engagement to develop "street cred" and to build trust is critical for the success of outbreak control, particularly in settings such as eastern DRC.

Greg Armstrong, director, Office of Advanced Molecular Detection Program, CDC, asked if the innovation of emergency operations centers has been helpful in improving timeliness and completeness of response, bringing partners together for better coordination, and giving governments a degree of engagement and control that they would not otherwise have. Bandyopadhyay replied that emergency operations centers have strengthened polio response efforts, especially in high-risk settings and in situations where response time is critical. They have also been used as platforms to build infrastructure and capacity to respond to other pathogens and threats, such as Ebola.

Cristina Cassetti, deputy division director, Division of Microbiology and Infectious Diseases, National Institute of Allergy and Infectious Diseases, asked if surveillance for acute flaccid paralysis during the polio eradication campaign also tests for related viruses that can cause paralysis, such as the enterovirus EV-D68. Bandyopadhyay replied that surveillance for acute flaccid paralysis partly involves clinical surveillance, with reporting based on symptoms of sudden-onset flaccidity in people aged less than 15 years, but it does include laboratory testing for nonpolio enteroviruses. Testing is categorized by whether a sample has polio, and if so, intratypic differentiation is conducted to classify whether it is wild or vaccine derived, which serotype it is, and if it contains nonpolio enteroviruses. They also do an ongoing assessment of nonpolio enterovirus prevalence in some of the settings, he added.

Keiji Fukuda, director and clinical professor, The University of Hong Kong School of Public Health, asked about the place of vaccine-associated polio phenomena within the overall goal of eradication. He suggested that political will and financing may dissipate for these polio campaigns. Bandyopadhyay emphasized the success of vaccination campaigns in reducing the number of wild cases outside of Afghanistan and Pakistan, although there are concerns that transmission is ongoing in those two countries. He reiterated that there is a conundrum around using the OPV. It is essential to interrupt transmission in the settings where a live vaccine is needed to provide intestinal immunity, but it is associated with risk in settings with consistently low immunization coverage.

He also expressed concern about the expanding nature of VDPVs, 90 percent of which are from the type 2 component of the virus, which is the component of the OPV that has been withdrawn from routine immunization use. He highlighted the global vulnerability around type 2 vaccine transmission. Outbreak response will need to be intensified using the available tools that can disrupt this transmission; but, at the same time, innovations are needed to develop improved vaccines with greater genetic stability. He added that a wild type 3 vaccine-derived outbreak would be concerning, but there are tools available to interrupt it if used effectively. Alternative tools are also under development that could solve the issue of seeding more vaccine-derived outbreaks, such as the novel OPV that is more genetically stable.

3

Harnessing Lessons from Emerging Scientific, Technological, and Social Innovations

The first session of the workshop aimed to harness lessons from emerging scientific, technological, and social innovations. The session's objective was to present case studies on the lessons learned from approaches that have enabled successful innovations for predictive modeling, big data, mobile health, and diagnostic and detection tools. The session was moderated by Greg Armstrong, director, Office of Advanced Molecular Detection, U.S. Centers for Disease Control and Prevention (CDC). Audrey Lenhart, lead, Insecticide Resistance and Vector Control Team, Center for Global Health/Division of Parasitic Diseases and Malaria Entomology Branch, CDC, explored the role of innovation in the evolution of global vector control response using the example of new vector control tools for malaria.

Caroline Buckee, associate director and associate professor, Center for Communicable Disease Dynamics, Department of Epidemiology at the Harvard T.H. Chan School of Public Health, presented on how new modeling approaches can be applied to inform infectious disease surveillance and outbreak response. Senjuti Saha, scientist, Child Health Research Foundation (CHRF), described the development of laboratory capacity for metagenomics sequencing to counter microbial threats in Bangladesh to explore the challenges and opportunities of developing this type of capacity in a lower-resource setting. Nitika Pant Pai, associate professor in the Department of Medicine, McGill University, examined the effect of digital process innovations for HIV self-testing on community-level health outcomes using evidence from Canada and South Africa.

THE ROLE OF INNOVATION IN THE EVOLUTION OF GLOBAL VECTOR CONTROL RESPONSE

Audrey Lenhart focused on malaria and the *Aedes*-borne arboviruses to explore the role of innovation in the evolution of global vector control response. These viruses represent the greatest public health burden globally among vector-borne diseases (WHO, 2017a). Malaria is a disease for which there is not currently a licensed vaccine, although chemoprophylaxis is available. As a result, efforts to prevent and control malaria rely heavily on control of the anopheles mosquito vectors. Traditionally, this has been accomplished through the use of insecticide-treated bed nets and the residual spraying of insecticides in houses. She explained that for the *Aedes*-born arboviruses—primarily dengue, Zika, and chikungunya—no widely licensed vaccines or chemotherapeutics are currently available. For these diseases, vector control is the only tool against both the adult mosquitoes and the aquatic stages of the mosquitoes. For both *Aedes* and *Anopheles* mosquito control, most traditional tools have the common denominator of heavy reliance on chemical insecticides. A consequence of this practice has been the widespread emergence of insecticide resistance in these mosquitoes.

Current State of Global Malaria Control Efforts

Insecticide resistance is a major threat to successful control of malaria and other *Aedes*- and *Anopheles*-borne diseases, said Lenhart. Despite the progress in malaria control seen in the early 2000s with the advent of large campaigns supported by The Global Fund to Fight AIDS, Tuberculosis and Malaria (The Global Fund) and the President's Malaria Initiative, progress has stagnated and stalled since 2015 (WHO, 2018a). Concurrently, the prevalence of insecticide resistance has increased in the vectors that transmit malaria. The global expansion of *Aedes*-borne arboviruses has driven an increase in vector control, with more insecticides being used to try to quell the outbreaks, which is also contributing to the emerging increase in the prevalence of insecticide resistance in these mosquitoes (Dusfour et al., 2019).

Lenhart explained that the World Health Organization (WHO) developed its global vector control response against this backdrop of stalled malaria control progress, continued reliance on insecticide-based interventions, and upward trends in insecticide resistance. Released in 2017, this strategic framework was designed to guide countries in how to address the growing threat of vector-borne diseases through 2030 (WHO, 2017a). She highlighted the framework's foundation, which calls for increases in basic and applied research, as well as innovations, to enable success in the four pillars of action (see Figure 3-1).

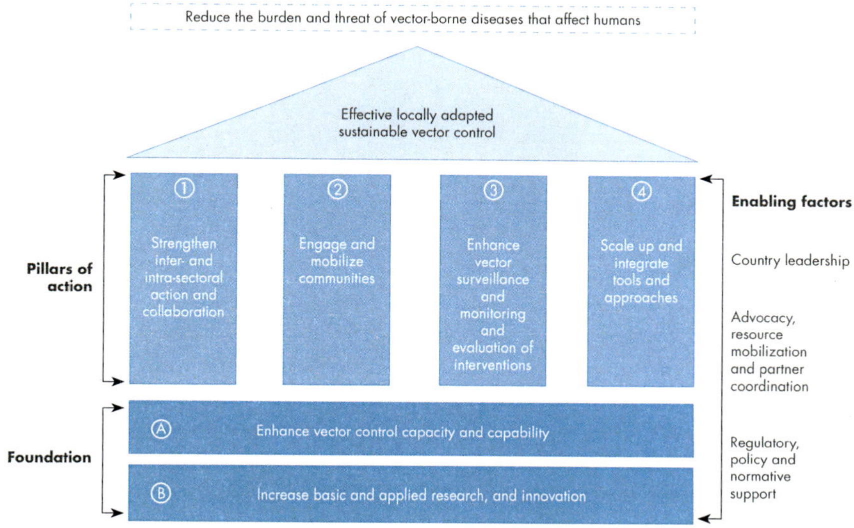

FIGURE 3-1 WHO's global vector control response framework.
SOURCES: Lenhart presentation, December 4, 2019; WHO, 2017a, 2019e.

Importance of Evidence-Based Innovations to Eliminate Malaria

Lenhart emphasized that because current vector control tools are insufficient, innovation is essential if malaria is to be eliminated. A modeling study summarized the fractions in decreases in childhood malaria attributable to insecticide-treated bed nets, indoor residual spraying of insecticides, and combination therapies; they found that though progress has been made, the impacts of these interventions are still below the elimination target (Bhatt et al., 2015). In addition to growing insecticide resistance, major gaps also exist around tools used to control outdoor-biting and day-biting vectors (*Aedes*), for example. She noted that innovations with the potential to address these gaps are currently under way, including new and repurposed insecticides with novel modes of action to which the mosquitoes are not yet resistant, noninsecticide-based strategies, and genetic modification.

An evidence base needs to be established for an innovation's effect, said Lenhart, because most large donor organizations will only procure vector control products that have a WHO recommendation. However, for WHO to make a policy recommendation on a vector control tool, it must demonstrate public health impact. WHO's Vector Control Advisory Group reviews evidence arising from trials with epidemiological endpoints in order to assess the public health impact of these vector control tools, she added. This process runs in parallel with the WHO prequalification process for vector control products, which assesses product efficacy, safety, and quality. The processes of bringing a new innovation into widespread use in donor-funded malaria control programs is challenging because it is lengthy and expensive, she added.

Lenhart described the New Nets Project as a case example of innovation in malaria control. The program is led by the Innovative Vector Control Consortium in partnership with The Global Fund and Unitaid. She described the Innovative Vector Control Consortium as an exemplar of innovation in the vector space because it was specifically created to foster innovation by convening partners from industry, the public sector, and academia in order to spur innovation for vector-borne disease tools. More information about the New Nets Project is provided in Box 3-1.

Many exciting new tools for vector control are in the pipeline, said Lenhart. She pointed out that controlling mosquitoes is not the sole concern: there must also be an impact on public health. Clinical trials have not traditionally been conducted to evaluate vector control tools. As a result, funding is scarce for generating the evidence base required to show the effect on public health. Procurement of innovative vector control tools is highly donor dependent, so the commercial market for these innovations is limited. This gives rise to the challenge of maintaining industry engagement in continued research and development of these tools. She added that the need for

BOX 3-1
Case Example of Innovation in Vector Control: New Nets Project

The New Nets Project was established with the parallel aims of building the evidence base required by the World Health Organization while conducting large-scale pilots of innovative tools. The project developed bed nets that contain novel combinations of insecticides, some of which have never previously been used for mosquito control. The project's objective is to assess the cost-effectiveness of these new innovative nets under large operational pilot conditions across countries representing an array of epidemiological insecticide resistance and entomological profiles. Millions of new nets are being distributed in numerous countries in Africa, including Burkina Faso, Côte d'Ivoire, Ghana, Liberia, Malawi, Mali, Mozambique, Nigeria, and Rwanda. Simultaneously, robustly designed cluster-randomized trials nested within the project are investigating the public health impact of these new nets. The project's team will negotiate the price reduction necessary to make the project sustainable, citing the large volumes procured during the pilot. The project also benefits from multisectoral collaboration among partners in industry, academia, implementing partners, and large-scale malaria initiatives.

SOURCES: Lenhart presentation, December 4, 2019; IVCC, n.d.

innovation will not dissipate in the future, because as mosquitoes continue to evolve so must the tools to control them.

APPLYING MODELING TO INFORM INFECTIOUS DISEASE SURVEILLANCE AND OUTBREAK RESPONSE

Caroline Buckee discussed the new sources of data being used to model disease outbreaks and the value of new, more complex mapping techniques that use these data in predictive models. She gave several examples of how these techniques and data have been used to model outbreaks in novel ways and direct the flow of resources, then described some of the barriers to broad implementation of these techniques and data. She explained that a new trend emerging in mathematical modeling for infectious diseases is the use of highly complex simulation models that appear to be detailed, accurate, and fit the data well. However, these models should not be embraced unless the data underlying them are accurate. She emphasized that a model is only as good as the data that underlie it.

Risk Mapping and Sources of Data

Buckee and her colleagues are working on the application of risk maps to improve the targeting of resources for infectious disease control. She explained that these risk maps are developed based on the incidence reports of clinical cases from hospitals and clinics around the country, and are used to allocate resources, which is especially important if resources are scarce. One challenge in using risk maps for resource allocation is the global increase in travel, including international travel; internal migration; and large-scale population displacement following natural disasters or conflicts. For example, if the size of a catchment area is assumed based solely on clinic reporting, then it is probably much larger than assumed. Another challenge Buckee noted is that long-term imported infections may appear to be happening in a specific place, but they will actually have a different point of origin. In the context of mathematical modeling, these dynamics need to be understood in order to help infectious disease control programs make decisions based on estimates of the speed at which a disease may spread out of a population at risk and the risk of importation to a population from an endemic area.

Buckee explained that from a modeling standpoint, epidemic numbers—such as the number of cases of Ebola in Sierra Leone—are plotted on a curve, which allows a simple mathematical model to be fit to the epidemic. This is done instead of using a statistical model because of the nonlinear dynamics that drive these types of outbreaks. Understanding that mechanism is necessary for interpreting the model parameter estimates, which are related to the epidemiological factors that underlie the spread, said Buckee. This elucidates the threshold conditions for reducing transmission and allows for evaluating the effectiveness of different interventions.

Most frameworks involve one population in an outbreak, but Buckee is interested in looking at spatial dynamics. Until recently, most models used some version of a gravity model for this purpose. Gravity models are developed from transportation theory and hold that large populations attract in a way that is inversely related to distance; that is, cities are attractors and places that are further away from cities have less travel (Haynes and Fotheringham, 1984). Although these models are analytically tractable, they are not validated, they do not have asymmetries in them, and they do not vary over time, Buckee noted.

New Sources of Data to Understand Real-Time Spatial Dynamics

An emerging approach is to work with new data sources to develop a better understanding of spatial dynamics in real time, said Buckee. These data sources can be used within epidemiological models to better understand the flow of disease over space and time. She noted that owing to the ubiquity of mobile phones, they can serve as a useful source of this information. Mobile operators already collect these data routinely, providing scalable information about the location and travel patterns of millions of people in nearly real time. To illustrate, she shared a data visualization demonstration that was developed in collaboration with Telenor, a Norwegian mobile operator, and their business unit in Bangladesh. The visualization tracked the population-wide travel from Dhaka, the capital of Bangladesh, to the countryside and back to Dhaka for the Eid holiday. It provides detailed information about the weekly dynamics of people's movements during that period. The use of these data raises concerns about privacy and data aggregation, requiring negotiation with national regulatory authorities to ensure that the data are secure. Efforts are under way to standardize these methods, she noted.

Other sources of data can be used to generate useful information about the spread of disease, said Buckee. For instance, Facebook, Google, and other companies are interested in developing their own methods of mapping population displacement and density to release routinely as well as during outbreaks and disasters. She suggested that these organizations should be engaged in a public forum around how privacy is handled in using these data, especially in the context of public health, because public perception will influence the effectiveness and impact of these approaches.

Combining Data Layers to Effectively Generate Useful Information

Modelers are working to bring together different types of data to target resources effectively to stop transmission of disease, Buckee said.

Traditional forms of epidemiological data on prevalence and incidence can be complemented by satellite information about vectorial capacity or the distribution in a village, for example, and mobile phone data and other kinds of information can provide more up-to-date population density estimates. Modelers need these data to determine the denominators for the population at risk, Buckee continued. Information about migration rates can be used to assess travel between regions and to inform estimates of importation and exportation in the spread of disease between regions. In the past, modelers were reliant on travel survey data, but they can now draw on other sources of information, such as mobile phone data and biological samples with genomic sequencing. Each of the data sources used in models has biases and problems associated with it, she explained. Therefore, the role of modelers is to bring these data together to make sense of the epidemiological situation.

She highlighted similarities between the emergence and the elimination of outbreaks, as shown in Figure 3-2. Both involve spatial heterogeneity. In emergence, researchers are seeking the early first cases of an outbreak; toward elimination, researchers are seeking the last cases of an outbreak. Some methods for these two efforts can translate between the two, although outbreak emergence calls for simpler modeling and faster communication.

Case Examples of Combination Modeling

Buckee presented examples of modeling work in which researchers used a combination of models and various sources of data to generate concrete outcomes. In Pakistan, researchers sought to move beyond a risk map for dengue fever, which shows the vectorial potential for transmission, and toward a targeted risk map that could predict whether Lahore will be at risk of dengue in 1 month, for example (Wesolowski et al., 2015). In Bangladesh, researchers combined models and data sources, including mobile phone and genetic data, to produce a map that estimated the fraction of cases in a particular region that were thought to be imported (Chang et al., 2019). Another project in which Buckee was involved worked with people on the ground in Mozambique just prior to Hurricane Kenneth. In response to concern about the spread of cholera, the project team conducted a simple modeling exercise to rapidly predict the areas at highest risk for cholera outbreak (Kahn et al., 2019). This exercise demonstrated the importance of strong organizational structure in achieving implementation, she said. They had a multisectoral, diverse, and flexible team that spanned the public sector, nongovernmental organizations, and academia; they were in continuous communication about what they needed to know and what data they had available.

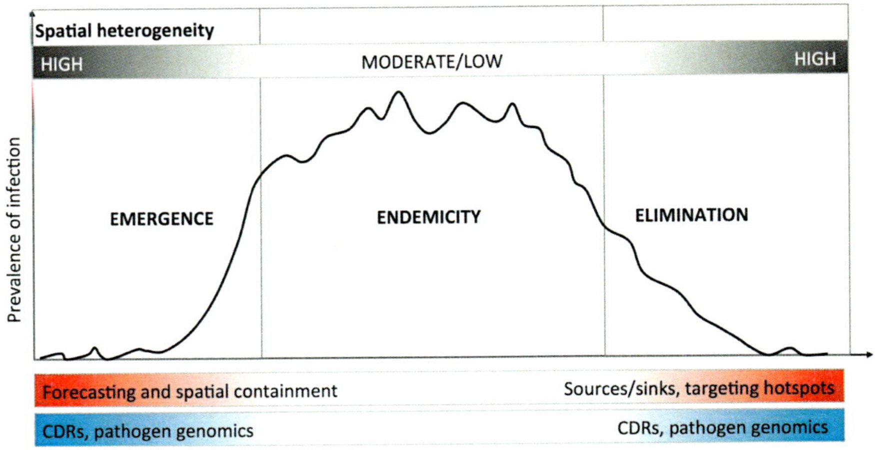

FIGURE 3-2 Optimal use of new approaches depends on epidemiological context.
NOTE: CDR = call data record.
SOURCES: Buckee presentation, December 4, 2019; Buckee et al., 2018.

Barriers to Translating Modeling Innovations to the Field

Buckee explored several barriers to translating innovations in modeling to the field. The first is that academic incentives are misaligned with translational goals. The incentives to write publications and secure grants are at odds with the translational goals of local capacity building, navigating regulatory and political issues, long-term engagement with infection control programs, and continuous methodological refinement. Regulatory and political issues are also restricting the feasibility of moving toward the use of private data for modeling. Academics are not well suited for the challenging and time-consuming process of negotiating data access, breaking down barriers between public and private stakeholders, and obtaining buy-in from relevant parties on the ground. She noted that even the best modeling approach will not be used to guide decision making if there is no demand for it or if the epidemiological data are weak. The quality of a model depends on quality reporting of epidemiological surveillance and response data, which is not prioritized in many cases, and on receiving feedback about which questions are most important to address.

Finally, she said that current funding mechanisms do not allow rapid response. Epidemic response requires responsive, flexible cross-sector teams that are in constant communication, rather than centralized hubs. These teams should be able to respond quickly, have domain area expertise, and be in close contact with epidemiologists on the ground—this is not typically possible for academics working within the constraints of large federal grants, for example. She added that surveillance work, including "peace time" methodological development, should be better integrated with teams that respond to crises.

UNBIASED METAGENOMICS SEQUENCING TO COUNTER MICROBIAL THREATS: LESSONS FROM BANGLADESH

Senjuti Saha described the development of a laboratory for metagenomic sequencing to counter microbial threats in Bangladesh to demonstrate the value of building capacity on site in countries that typically outsource this type of work. She explained that CHRF's mission is to improve the evidence needed to inform policy decisions that would improve child health in Bangladesh and around the world. To aid policy makers in making data-driven decisions, CHRF established a pathogen surveillance program in Bangladesh that is carried out in microbiology laboratories in four hospitals across the country, with support from WHO Rotavirus and Invasive Bacterial Vaccine Preventable Diseases Sentinel hospital sites.

The objectives of the pathogen surveillance program in Bangladesh are (1) to describe the etiology, the epidemiology, and the burden of diseases, including meningitis, sepsis, pneumonia, and enteric fever; (2) to establish a platform to measure vaccine needs and impact; and (3) to characterize circulating pathogen types, including antimicrobial resistance and serotypes. CHRF has maintained a focus on four priority pathogens: *Neisseria meningitidis*, *Streptococcus pneumoniae*, *Haemophilus influenzae* type b (Hib), and group B *Streptococcus*.

Collaborating to Develop Local Capacity for Metagenomic Sequencing

Saha's presentation focused on meningitis sequencing in Dhaka Shishu Hospital, the largest pediatric hospital in the country. In 1993, CHRF began surveillance using culture to detect the etiology of meningitis in cerebrospinal fluid, gradually adding serology and antigen testing and progressing from conventional polymerase chain reaction (PCR) to quantitative PCR (qPCR) in 2015. In spite of their extensive efforts, the etiology of many meningitis cases remains unknown. Between 2003 and 2016, Saha remarked that the hospital collected 24,000 samples of cerebral spinal fluid, including 8,000 cases of suspected infectious meningitis based on ≥ 10 white blood cells per cubic millimeter, a biomarker of clinical meningitis. Even among cases where the white blood cell count was more than 500, researchers were unable to determine the etiology in more than half of those cases. This lack of evidence hampered efforts to institute data-driven policies for prevention or treatment, she noted.

The group at CHRF hypothesized that RNA metagenomics could solve the mystery, but they had no evidence to show that they could conduct even the simplest sequencing on site in the hospital's small laboratory. Typically, this kind of research is done remotely by a country in the Global North, which does not build capacity in Bangladesh. In 2018, CHRF was able to break this cycle by developing capacity for metagenomic sequencing through a collaboration with the Chan Zuckerberg Biohub. The Biohub had expertise in solving cases of meningitis with unknown etiology, and the hospital had years of samples with case-based electronic data. To ensure that the collaboration was bilaterally beneficial, they ensured that all standard operating procedures were open access, all technologies and pipelines resulting from the collaboration were transferrable and sustainable, local scientists would be trained through the collaboration, and the local group would own the data produced through the collaboration.

Elucidating the Causative Agents of Meningitis Using Metagenomics

Saha provided an overview of the collaboration to elucidate the causative agents of meningitis using metagenomics. During the first phase, 96 samples were collected and sent to the Biohub laboratories in San Francisco: 36 positive controls that were etiology-confirmed using standard laboratory techniques in Bangladesh; 36 negative controls that were noninfectious cases of meningitis and water samples; and 25 "mystery" idiopathic cases, in which etiology could not be attributed using standard laboratory techniques. They extracted RNA from all of the samples, prepared a library, and then sequenced and analyzed the samples.

She noted that the most challenging process was analyzing the vast amount of data culled from each sample. To assist with analysis, the collaborators used the free, open source software IDSeq that has useful embedded software called "Background," which helps to control for environmental RNA contaminants in different settings. They used the negative control samples to establish the microbial distribution that is normally present everywhere. Using that as a background, they gave every pathogen in the positive and idiopathic samples a Z score. Based on the Z score, they were able to model any pathogens that were found.

Her team found high concordance among the positive and negative controls, said Saha (Saha et al., 2019a). When pathogens were found using metagenomics and their model, there was a high likelihood that it was a true pathogen. However, pathogens that were found using qPCR with very high cycle threshold values tended to be missed by metagenomics. They did not find any significant pathogens in their negative control samples. Idiopathic samples were found to contain a diverse range of pathogens, she reported. Out of 25 idiopathic samples tested, 10 were solved by the metagenomic analysis (Saha et al., 2019a). Saha pointed out that these samples were not collected or stored with the intention of analyzing them with a sensitive method such as metagenomics. Clinical follow-up of the 10 cases that were solved by metagenomic analysis revealed three cases of chikungunya, which is a relatively new virus in Bangladesh (Saha et al., 2019a). They were aware that the virus causes fevers, but they did not realize that it was crossing the blood–brain barrier and causing chikungunya meningitis.

Further investigation revealed that these three cases originated during the first large chikungunya outbreak in Bangladesh in summer 2017. The researchers suspected that there were more cases of chikungunya that had been missed, but they could not afford to conduct unbiased metagenomics on hundreds of samples. Instead, they optimized a low-cost qPCR method to test almost 500 stored cerebral spinal fluid samples from 2017. Using this method, they discovered that 12 percent of all meningitis cases that came into the hospital that summer were positive for chikungunya. By comparing these findings with cases of chikungunya fever recorded during the same time period, Saha and her colleagues showed that there had been an undocumented chikungunya meningitis outbreak that overlapped with the chikungunya fever outbreak in summer 2017 (Saha et al., 2019a). The success of this effort allowed the researchers to secure funding for the second phase of the project, during which they transferred the technology to Bangladesh and set up a small metagenomics laboratory.

Developing Local Sequencing Capacity: Barriers and Opportunities

Saha described some of the challenges involved in setting up a sequencing platform laboratory in a low- and middle-income country (LMIC) such as Bangladesh. For instance, it is difficult to obtain supplies because distributors and manufacturers do not have local offices in Bangladesh, which requires laboratories to work with resellers or local distributors to obtain reagents. These distributors tend to charge higher prices for local laboratories, she noted. In this case, Saha's colleagues in San Francisco were able to negotiate on behalf of the laboratory in Bangladesh to help them obtain supplies at a lower cost. However, without such intervention, small laboratories in lower-income settings lack the power or influence to negotiate for fair pricing. Laboratories in LMICs must also deal with infrastructure issues, she added. For example, Dhaka is a very hot city with poor air quality, which requires setting up equipment to control temperature, humidity, and dust content.

Saha maintained that these challenges are all surmountable with the help of global collaboration and the enthusiasm of local scientists in the laboratory to participate in this research (Saha et al., 2018, 2019b). Her team has been able to empower, educate, and engage local scientists on the front lines of public health. Furthermore, this work built the capacity in Dhaka to use metagenomics to investigate the severe outbreak of dengue fever in 2019, which affected more than 100,000 people with high rates of mortality, by sequencing cerebral spinal fluid and serum samples in real time. The lab is also using metagenomics for nationwide mosquito surveillance for dengue fever, chikungunya, and Zika in order to help predict outbreaks and outbreak severity.

Much progress is being made, Saha noted, but this is just the beginning of a long-term process that is being undertaken by CHRF. In 2018, CHRF staff performed 3,000 cultures on blood from children who were suspected of having sepsis. At that time, researchers were able to attribute etiology to only 17 percent of these samples, and all of those patients were treated with antibiotics—which probably included third-generation cephalosporins. This speaks to the magnitude of the "unknowns" that Saha and her colleagues at CHRF are working to address. She closed by encouraging a more holistic approach to outbreak investigation. Rather than using an etiology-by-etiology approach, she suggested using methods between endemics to build landscapes or maps of known pathogens in order to detect emerging and reemerging outbreaks.

DIGITAL PROCESS INNOVATIONS FOR HIV SELF-TESTING

Nitika Pant Pai presented on how digital process innovations for HIV self-testing can affect health outcomes at the community level, drawing on experiences in South Africa and Canada. She explained that HIV self-testing is a self-screening process whereby end users perform the test on their own by collecting their own blood or oral samples, interpreting and recording their test results, and proactively seeking linkages to counseling and care. The U.S. Food and Drug Administration (FDA) approved the first in-home, oral HIV self-test in 2012 (FDA, 2014). Four years later, WHO released guidelines on HIV self-testing and partner notification stating that self-testing could complement conventional testing strategies, particularly in the last mile of care (WHO, 2016). As of 2019, more than 70 countries had HIV self-testing guidelines or policies in place (WHO, 2019d). HIV self-testing has been implemented as part of the effort to end the HIV epidemic, she noted.

Overview of the HIVSmart! App

HIVSmart! is an app-based program designed with support from the McGill University Health Centre and the Government of South Africa to help people in LMICs self-test their own HIV status, said Pant Pai. The program addresses several gaps in efforts to achieve the targets set forth in 2014 by the Joint United Nations Programme on HIV/AIDS to end the HIV epidemic, which are known as the 90-90-90 targets. These targets call for 90 percent of all people living with HIV to know their HIV status by 2020, ensuring that 90 percent of those diagnosed with HIV receive treatment by 2020, and viral suppression of 90 percent of all people receiving antiretroviral therapy by 2020 (UNAIDS, 2014). Although HIV self-testing has expanded access, she noted, it is unclear how well the self-tests are being administered. Other concerns relate to interpreting and storing the test results, ensuring timely linkages from self-testing to counseling and care, and keeping patients in care (Pant Pai et al., 2013a). Pant Pai explained that HIVSmart! has evolved from an app to a complete program of care that provides an efficient method of screening, counseling, and treatment for patients and providers. The program offers the following multiple services delivered in tandem:

- Evidence-based HIV information;
- A user-friendly, language tailored, mobile app;
- Step-by-step instructions for self-test conduct;
- Pretest risk assessment and counseling;
- Rapid self-test results;
- Secure and confidential cloud storage of data;
- Geolocations of clinics for confirmatory testing;
- 24/7 counseling in multiple forms; and
- Rapid linkages to antiretroviral therapy and retention in care.

Evidence for App-Based HIV Self-Testing

Pant Pai presented some of the evidence that has accrued to support app-based HIV self-testing with HIVSmart! The program was initially a web-based HIV self-testing strategy, piloted by university students in Canada in 2009 (Pant Pai et al., 2014) and by health care workers in South Africa (Pant Pai et al., 2013b); the app-based version of HIVSmart! was initially tested in Montreal with a cross-sectional study (Pant Pai et al., 2018). Between 2016 and 2018, the app-based HIVSmart! program was evaluated among 3,000 people in South African townships using an observational cohort study design to see if it would help people actually conduct self-testing, seek linkages to care, and receive treatment (Janssen et al., 2020).

Pant Pai explained that in process innovation, cohort study designs have advantages over randomized controlled trials in that they can capture how participants receive the innovation as well as the dimension of choice and other conceptual underpinnings that determine how participants integrate the innovation into their lives. Participants in the study were given a choice between two popular self-testing strategies: (1) supervised self-testing, whereby individuals conduct the self-test in the presence of a health care professional in a clinic setting, and (2) unsupervised self-testing, whereby individuals obtain self-tests from a pharmacy and conduct the self-test at home (Janssen et al., 2020). The second strategy is more common in the United States, she noted.

The study investigated how people chose between these two strategies and how they integrated the self-tests into their lives. It also explored the effects of these strategies on linkages to care, on the detection of new infections, and on the expansion of access to care. The study provided participants with the HIVSmart! app on their phones; half of the 1,500 participants chose the supervised strategy and the others chose the unsupervised strategy, she reported. During the rollout of this program, some participants reported that they did not have enough space in their homes to safely conduct the self-testing strategy and requested that a kiosk be set up near the clinic where they could safely conduct the self-test without supervision. She noted that this is an example of how an innovation can be tailored to setting-specific needs.

Almost all of the participants returned for care; some participants returned to the clinic setting while others wanted to return to clinics outside of the setting. The geolocation feature of the HIVSmart! app allowed researchers to monitor where participants were seeking linkages to care and to connect with participants and ensure that almost all of them receive care. The intervention also expanded access to care, she added. HIV self-testing through the app became so popular among the community that they were able to discontinue the social media campaign advertising its benefits.

Challenges and Opportunities in HIV Self-Testing Strategies

Pant Pai described some of the challenges encountered in implementing HIV self-testing strategies. Connectivity issues were common, and some participants had smartphones that were not able to fully use the functionality of the HIVSmart! app. This was resolved by allowing these participants to either use the supervised strategy or to implement the unsupervised strategy in one of the offsite kiosks. It was also challenging to mobilize care seeking outside of clinics. Health Insurance Portability and Accountability Act compliance required the use of firewalls that were challenging to address. The app was also met with resistance based on skepticism of new technology. Some people rejected the app, for example, because they thought the digital innovation would be detrimental by undermining peer navigators that were already in place in the health care system. Pant Pai worked to build confidence in the system among health care providers and patients, who eventually requested that the program be rolled out community-wide.

To address other challenges at the outset, Pant Pai's team customized the app to the context and made it culturally adaptable, so they were able to work around language issues. To address ethical considerations, the qualitative component of the cohort study explored the tension between autonomy and risk mitigation—that is, between wanting privacy and negotiating presence (Janssen et al., 2020). The participants reported that they most appreciated the ability to negotiate their space, their level of support, and the testing process itself. They also liked the fact that the process was simple and confidential and that they could self-determine where, with whom, and when to self-test. In the context of future opportunities, Pant Pai noted that the HIVSmart! strategy has been adopted by Fast-Track Cities with support from the International Association of Providers of AIDS Care. Pant Pai's team is working to customize the strategy for use in Canada and hopes to scale up this strategy for other key populations and hotspots to help eliminate HIV.

DISCUSSION

Carolyn Carroll asked how Buckee was able to persuade Telenor to provide data, given existing privacy concerns. Buckee responded that she has worked with multiple mobile operators in this space of research for some time, and Telenor has taken the lead in the industry in terms of finding ways to use their data for public health and other socially beneficial projects. She explained that Telenor has its own research group working on how to use its data for these projects within its multilevel privacy and security process that works with business units, regulators, and governments to ensure that data stay within the operator in-country. Aggregated matrices are sent to the research group in Oslo, which then shares the data with select academic researchers.

Buckee pointed out that the data are provided at such a large scale that the information is memoryless and aggregated to many towers at once; it does not reveal information about individual trajectories, and reidentification of individuals is not possible after the aggregate data are shared. She noted that the creation of these types of aggregations for different purposes has been a matter of concern, but Telenor has been at the forefront of making sure it is done safely. Buckee confirmed that reidentification of individuals is impossible through Telenor's processes prior to providing the data.

Eva Harris, director, Center for Global Public Health, University of California, Berkeley, asked Lenhart about community involvement in the New Nets Project. Lenhart explained that she is not part of the New Nets Project, but the communities receiving nets through the program are not doing so for the first time; they are receiving innovative replacement nets treated with dual insecticide. She added that within any of these large initiatives, there are community engagement components, particularly around the potential misuse of bed nets.

Harris asked Buckee about issues with data sharing—such as funder requirements to make the deidentified data available for public analysis—that might dissuade local stakeholders from putting in time to collect the data for other people to analyze. She also flagged the work required to harmonize and apply standards to data analysis, noting a tension between the Global North, where people may like data to be publicly available for analysis, and the people collecting the data in the Global South, where people collecting the data may want to control how they are used or analyzed. Buckee remarked that the incentive structures within academia can be pernicious in that people collecting data often fail to receive the authorship and credit they deserve, for example. She noted that there is a similar glamorization of the analytics and artificial intelligence (AI) in modeling, while the work of actually collecting highly detailed epidemiological data is less appreciated. She called for a shift in the academic world to frame global health research as unlike other branches of science. In terms of data sharing, another issue is the pressure for countries to share all of their epidemiological data. Although this is framed as being in their best interests regionally and globally, some countries may not be eager to do so.

Marcos Espinal, director, Department of Communicable Diseases and Environmental Determinants of Health, Pan American Health Organization, applauded Buckee's call for people to be put first and accounted for by policy makers in order for modeling to be helpful. Espinal put modeling in the context of human movement and migration, which is often politicized as being damaging rather than beneficial. He noted that policy makers sometimes use modeling results for predicting an outbreak in a certain place as an excuse to deport migrants.

Espinal offered the example of Venezuelan migrants to Colombia, Ecuador, and Peru being blamed for bringing in diseases such as malaria, giving rise to serious human rights issues. Buckee added that policy makers' responses often depend on which level of government they are in; for example, in a national malaria control program, policy makers may be less interested in blaming people and more interested in trying to control the disease. She noted that public perception of new modeling approaches at the community level, which are often shaped by Facebook and other social media platforms, can be the most hostile.

In terms of higher levels of government, Buckee said, one of the things modeling has shown is that shutting a border down to keep out migrants will not stop an epidemic. This is an outdated idea based on migration patterns from 100 years ago, Buckee said. She suggested that models and data demonstrate that the world is globally connected, but scientists have not sufficiently demonstrated the value of that connectedness. In infectious disease outbreaks, notions of national identity are blurred and inconsequential with respect to pathogen transmission. She pointed out that feedback from policy makers also depends on their level in a government. For instance, policy makers at lower levels may not wish to be perceived as tied up with corporate interests. For policy makers at higher levels of government, Buckee proposed treating epidemics as a global issue. She suggested focusing on building lab capacity in LMICs and helping governments and ministries of health build the capacity to manage epidemics.

Tom Scott, director and professor, Department of Entomology, University of California, Davis, asked about the development and application of innovation in two areas: the first phase of coming up with an idea and carrying it through to the proof of principle to build up an evidence base, and the second phase of scaling it up to delivery of appropriate coverage in order to achieve the desired public health outcome. Scott asked about the challenges and barriers encountered in each respective phase and about issues related to delivering at scale that occur despite the innovation of ideas and work to complete proof of principle.

Pant Pai responded that universities and granting agencies are supporting innovation, but the support systems needed to scale an innovation are not in place. Pant Pai said that training in science, epidemiology, and medicine equips researchers to prove that an innovation works scientifically; however, businesses use the approach of releasing innovations and allowing the market to improve on it through an iterative approach of failing and learning. She noted that scaling up requires liaising with different stakeholders who need to share the intent of ensuring that innovations reach the people in need and suggested setting up a coalition among agencies that can support academics, scientists, and innovators in scaling interventions for the greater good. Pant Pai remarked that the current academic system's focus on publishing makes universities less likely to support innovations that are for the greater good, which will need to be addressed in order to make progress.

Saha added that the discussion around innovation and scaling interventions highlights the issue of power imbalance, because many innovations driven by donors and research agendas are meaningless if they are not implemented where they are needed most. However, better coordination will be needed to scale up innovations, she said. For example, WHO's Invasive Bacterial Vaccine-Preventable Diseases Laboratory Network, which spans approximately 150 laboratories in more than 50 countries and operates alongside WHO networks for the flu and rotavirus, do not communicate with each another (WHO, 2017b). Saha called for these actors to coordinate with one another to scale up interventions by leveraging existing infrastructure, rather than building parallel systems.

Buckee added that there is too much emphasis on innovation and pilot projects that only last for 1 year, which is not long enough to achieve meaningful results. She suggested moving away from rewarding innovation and focusing on scaling and implementation, which is more difficult and requires creative thinking. She noted that innovation in public health requires constant investment and evaluation, while innovation in the private sector tends to take off when the market drives it. Pant Pai said focusing on implementation and scale up will require aligning funds and bringing together cross-sector expertise to scale up innovations.

Daniel Berman, lead, Longitude Prize, remarked that Pant Pai made a strong case from the user perspective that HIVSmart! was making a difference in people seeking to know their HIV status. He asked for more information about the number of patients who have undetectable levels of the virus, the percentage of patients who say that they are staying on treatment, and transmission rates. Berman also stated that the system in South Africa is stronger than in other settings, but there are still disruptions to the supply of antiretrovirals that lead to increases in transmission rates and patients getting sick again because drugs are not available. Berman asked if issues such as medicine disruptions or clinic closures could be tracked through the app to help the system to serve its patients better.

Pant Pai said that she only focused on linkage and retention, but the app could potentially be expanded to connect geolocation hotspots and use machine learning to predict outcomes. Pant Pai said that these types of innovations seem in line with the South African government's focus on simple solutions and the use of technology. Berman added that the process of scaling up extends beyond academic institutions, and that private companies or nonprofit organizations could possibly use surveillance data that expose flaws in health systems that cannot be used by governments, owing to their potential political volatility.

4

Overcoming Barriers in the Field to Bolster Access and Practical Use of Innovations

The second session of the workshop focused on overcoming barriers in the field to bolster access and practical use of innovations. The session's objective was to elucidate the key barriers and facilitators to implementing innovative approaches that empower end users and patients, facilitate positive behavior change, and ultimately reduce the health impact of infectious diseases at the community level. The session was moderated by Eva Harris, director, Center for Global Public Health, University of California, Berkeley. Collince Osewe, founder and chief executive officer, ChanjoPlus, described how ChanjoPlus empowers health workers to improve immunization service delivery through digital innovation. Brian Bird, research virologist, One Health Institute, University of California, Davis, discussed the translation of data and modeling insights into improved capacity for detection and response using examples from his work following the outbreak of Ebola in West Africa. Carolina dos S. Ribeiro, senior policy advisor, Centre for Infectious Disease Control, the Netherlands, discussed issues related to global data sharing and collaboration and suggested a set of practical tools to enhance the timely sharing of outbreak data. Fadi Makki, founder, Nudge Lebanon and the Consumer Citizen Lab, described the application of insights from behavioral sciences to enhance acceptability and adoption of innovations across diverse social and cultural contexts.

DIGITAL INNOVATION TO IMPROVE IMMUNIZATION SERVICE DELIVERY

Collince Osewe presented on how health workers can be empowered to improve immunization service delivery through digital innovation. He described how he drew on his experience as a community health volunteer in Kenya to develop the ChanjoPlus mobile app to support the equitable delivery of vaccines at the community level. In Kenya and other countries in Africa, immunization management and reporting are still manual, paper-based processes. Community health workers visit households to identify underimmunized children and refer them to health facilities. This process typically depends on immunization booklets, which contain a child's vaccination history and must be updated every time a mother brings the child to a health facility. These booklets serve as the source documents for the entire immunization reporting structure. He explained that this manual process does not provide real-time visibility of performance and contributes to poor disease surveillance and inconsistencies in reporting.

He noted that Africa faces a substantial burden of underimmunization of children: an estimated 19 million children across the continent are underimmunized, and nearly one-fifth of children have not had all basic vaccinations (WHO, 2019f). He added that these factors contribute to a disease burden of $5 billion (Ozawa et al., 2017).

Empowering Health Workers and Improving Service Delivery with the Platform

Osewe described some of the challenges facing health workers in countries in Africa. The new generation of health workers frequently relocates, because there are multiple facilities offering the same spectrum of services. They conduct their work in the context of poor data, limited visibility, and ineffective vaccination tracking tools. Medical facilities are often fragmented and do not share their data with one another. To help address some of these challenges, ChanjoPlus was developed as a decentralized mobile health platform that allows health workers to access a centralized database of immunization status information. The platform does not require a smartphone or Internet and helps health workers to accurately identify children and their immunization records. With this information, they can track children who miss vaccines, and improve immunization data for real-time monitoring.

Community health volunteers register children by dialing the code into a mobile phone and using the platform to capture the child's demographic information and update the child's immunization status. Each child is assigned to the identification number of an adult within the household. During routine immunization services, a community volunteer can validate the adult's identity and then view the vaccines that each child in the household has received, as well as any vaccines that have been missed. The community health care worker has credentials to determine which vaccines to administer and then uses the platform to update a child's vaccine status. Once immunization updates are captured, they are available on the real-time immunization performance monitoring dashboard, which is accessible to the Ministry of Health.

Osewe described the benefits of this type of simple technological innovation. ChanjoPlus has been able to increase accountability for immunization resources and help to prevent waste and shortages, because real-time data can be used to determine the demand level in each facility and region. The platform also offers population-wide analytics on immunization and vaccinations in real time. In addition to improving data quality and verifiability, it can improve the efficiency of health workers because it provides immediate access to a child's immunization status, reducing service delivery times from 30 minutes to less than 5 minutes. He added that ChanjoPlus has also been found to reduce the cost of vaccination by approximately 47 percent, from \$7.00 per child to \$2.50 per child. ChanjoPlus is suitable for scale up across low-resource settings in sub-Saharan Africa, said Osewe. The platform has already been successfully piloted with about 14,000 children, and scale up is planned to 100,000 children in western Kenya during 2020.

Adoption and Sustainability of the Platform

Osewe described the challenges that ChanjoPlus has encountered while piloting the program in Kenya. Many organizations are working on innovation, but there is not a controlled environment for determining which innovations should be scaled up. ChanjoPlus is competing with large international companies that are entering the space with competing apps and innovations, rather than working with local stakeholders to develop in-country solutions. ChanjoPlus's path to adoption and sustainability relies on partnerships with implementers as well as partners who inform policy and uptake, he noted. ChanjoPlus has an incentivized cadre of volunteers that benefits from the currently devolved function of health care in Kenya: community health volunteers are recognized as part of the health care workforce and paid by the Kenyan government. He remarked that ChanjoPlus adds value across the value chain, from efficiency in service delivery to tracking children who need vaccinations to data analytics. He attributed the adoption of the platform to his company's human-centered design approach that engaged with mothers and health care workers, who voiced their challenges and offered solutions in the design of the platform. To ensure sustainability, they are seeking government uptake by framing the platform as a cost-reduction strategy delivered through a subscription model.

USING DATA AND MODELING TO IMPROVE DETECTION AND RESPONSE

Brian Bird explored how data and modeling insights can be translated into improved capacity for detection and response by reflecting on lessons learned during the West Africa Ebola outbreak and the work of the U.S. Agency for International Development's (USAID's) PREDICT project. He focused on community engagement, describing the local community as the grassroots stakeholder that can serve as the greatest facilitator as well as a potential barrier to successful implementation of a One Health approach to disease surveillance and supporting public health on a global scale. One Health zoonotic disease surveillance methods are critical for early outbreak detection and response, he maintained.

Lessons from the West Africa Ebola Virus Outbreak

Although he had worked on other filovirus outbreaks, the West Africa Ebola outbreak was an eye-opening experience for Bird. From 2013 to 2016, waves of human-to-human transmission led to more than 28,000 cases of Ebola and 11,000 deaths in West Africa. Past outbreaks had been smaller and less complex, with community relations built around a single village or country. However, when an outbreak expands into multiple countries and linguistic environments, community relations can quickly spiral out of control and it is impossible to respond effectively if communities do not trust emergency response teams.

Bird emphasized that the public health, One Health, and global health cadres are failing to scientifically communicate their messages in clear, concise ways that people can understand. He noted that poor community trust and engagement coupled with a lack of understanding of communities' fundamental motivations and beliefs stymied detection and control efforts during the Ebola outbreak in West Africa. For example, the personal protective equipment worn by researchers during an outbreak response can be frightening and intimidating to communities. Furthermore, the concepts of disease causation do not necessarily exist for people in Sierra Leone, who tend to have a more holistic construct of the world that does not encompass things such as microbes that cannot be seen, making it challenging to explain viral diseases to people in order to prevent transmission. To address this challenge, they used hand-drawn picture-books created by local artists as information-conveying tools in Sierra Leone to explain how to prevent Ebola transmission.

Adding further complexity, proper preparations of corpses for burial are required to control Ebola, but in West Africa, burial practices are intense community efforts that can lead to infectious corpses becoming powerful vectors of transmission. In one instance, 75 cases of Ebola were attributed to a single infectious corpse. The active inclusion of traditional healers and leaders in response efforts helped to change practices to allow for medically "safe and dignified burials" to break transmission chains. Unfortunately, community-level resistance and mistrust remained. He added that without careful attention, these types of issues will impede the deployment of any innovative, enhanced detection or response efforts.

PREDICT Surveillance Program and the PREDICT Ebola Host Project

Bird explained that the PREDICT project, funded by USAID, emerged from efforts during the Ebola outbreak in West Africa. The project was developed to perform global surveillance for emerging viral pathogens at the key interfaces between wildlife reservoirs, domestic animals, and people. It aimed to conduct One Health surveillance in real time while looking for novel emerging pandemic threats across a spectrum of transmission: virus evolution, cross-species transmission, animal-to-human spillover, human-to-human transmission, and international spread. PREDICT was a global project, operating in more than 30 countries in Africa and Asia between 2016 and 2019, that strengthened training and capacity building in these regions.[1]

Within the broader PREDICT program, Bird explained that the PREDICT Ebola Host Project (EHP) was launched with three core objectives: (1) to identify the animal origins of the Ebola virus; (2) to increase capacity for One Heath disease surveillance, including field sampling, laboratory, and behavior assessment; and (3) to work hand in hand with local communities, traditional leaders, and governments.

PREDICT EHP was established in Guinea, Liberia, and Sierra Leone—the three countries most severely affected by the West Africa Ebola outbreak—to conduct an in-depth, high-volume, high-intensity animal sampling to find the elusive reservoir of the Zaire Ebola virus, which was the causative agent of the West Africa outbreak as well as the more recent cases in the Democratic Republic of the Congo.

Outcomes of the PREDICT Project

Bird said that the project did not find the reservoir of the virus, although a bat infected with what looks like Ebola Zaire was found in Liberia. However, PREDICT EHP did achieve other substantial gains. Working hand in hand with traditional leaders and government structures, they were able to bring scientific information and capacity training down to as close to the village level as possible. The EHP teams included government representatives, vet-

[1] More information on the PREDICT project can be found at https://ohi.vetmed.ucdavis.edu/programs-projects/predict-project/about (accessed March 3, 2020).

erinary and medical surveillance officers, and laboratory technicians. They were able to sample a wide variety of environments, ecosystems, and species across the three countries in one of the largest in-depth biodiversity surveys ever done in West Africa. Bird noted that PREDICT EHP sampled 19,800 animals—primarily bats, because they had been less studied in the region. They trained 250 people in various One Health skills, including laboratory and surveillance skills, and worked in 60 communities across the region.

He said that each of these communities was provided risk-avoidance information and materials, and the EHP team worked with these communities to deeply engage them and help them understand the work being done. To do so, each team explained to the community members that they were searching for the source of the virus that may have killed loved ones within that community. Although PREDICT EHP did not find Ebola Zaire, the teams' work at the reservoir taxa level enabled them to find an entirely new species of Ebola virus, the Bombali virus, which raised the species count from five to six (Forbes et al., 2019; Goldstein et al., 2018). This was the first discovery of an Ebola virus that had not yet caused a known human or animal death. The co-discovery of Marburg virus in bats occurred almost simultaneously, he added (CDC, 2018). Marburg virus is a known killer of humans in central, eastern, and southern Africa, so the discovery of the virus 3,000 kilometers due west had significant public health implications (CDC, 2018).

PREDICT Project Successes and Lessons Learned

Bird outlined some of the lessons learned from the PREDICT project, as well as factors that made the project successful. The project used an innovative, integrated approach to finding viruses that highlights the "unknowns" about what to do next to manage risks (e.g., it is not yet known whether the Bombali virus is a human pathogen because it was found in a reservoir species). It is important to explain these types of discoveries in an appropriate way to policy makers and others, he noted. For instance, PREDICT EHP personnel worked hand in hand with the government of Sierra Leone to shape consistent and noninflammatory public messaging after the new viruses were discovered; extensive local public engagement reduced fear and misinformation.

The EHP team developed trust as they continuously collected samples in communities for several years and returned to communities to report the discovery of the two viruses, including one that is a high-risk public health pathogen and the other that is of unknown pathogenicity. Having built high trust with the community allowed for open and honest discussion about risks, he said. For example, the Bombali virus was found in a bat that often lives in the houses of community members—it is difficult to explain that Ebola has been found in a bat in a person's house, but that the risk is not yet known. Scientific work is needed to develop strategies to convey those types of messages, he said.

The PREDICT project demonstrates that overcoming trust barriers is necessary to save lives and that integrated One Health approaches paired with in-country governments do work, said Bird. Researchers should maintain a consistent presence in communities, working in partnership with community members, and convey scientific information in a way that people understand and accept. "The best next-generation diagnostic tools will not be of any benefit if people are reluctant to come to the clinic," he said, emphasizing that the ability of communities to augment response efforts should not be underestimated.

OUTBREAK-RELATED DATA SHARING AND COLLABORATION: CHALLENGES AND OPPORTUNITIES

Carolina dos S. Ribeiro examined issues related to the global practices of sharing microbial and genetic data during outbreaks. She also explored strategies for fostering collaboration and enhancing timely data sharing to tackle microbial threats.

Lessons from Recent Epidemic Responses

Ribeiro explained that recent global health crises caused by emerging infectious diseases, from Middle East respiratory syndrome (MERS) through Ebola to Zika, have revealed fundamental challenges in collaboration and data sharing that have affected epidemic investigation, national and international response, and the affected communities. For instance, the 2012 MERS epidemic in the Middle East highlighted issues of data ownership. The Saudi government strongly opposed a foreign patent on the virus sequence used to develop diagnostic tests on the grounds of protecting their sovereignty and national interests, thus restricting the sharing of virus materials and data from the outset of the epidemic. She noted that as a zoonotic disease with camels as a source of infection, MERS required a strong integrated response at the human–animal interface under the One Health approach. Instead, there was strong denial of animal involvement from the camel livestock sector and late engagement of animal health authorities (Keegan, 2014).

During the 2014 Ebola epidemic in West Africa, there were gaps in data sharing even when the number of cases was peaking (Yozwiak et al., 2015). No new virus sequences were released between August 2 and November 9 of that year, which was the period in which the largest number of new cases were discovered (Yozwiak et al., 2015). Genome sequences were shared only sporadically, even though more were known to have been generated. She added that research, response, and data sharing were uncoordinated and misaligned with the public health and decision-making needs of the national governments. She described the 2015 Zika epidemic as a clear example of government and regulatory restrictions on the international sharing of pathogen materials and data (Cheng et al., 2016; Koopmans et al., 2019). An external consortium initiative worked to develop external quality assurance and validation for Zika diagnostics, but after 1 year, only three laboratories had managed to complete all of the steps. Although this delay was primarily attributable to the lack of capacity and shipping materials, noted Ribeiro, the need to obtain government permission was also time consuming.

Data-sharing issues extend beyond outbreak timelines, said Ribeiro. In February 2019, for example, *The Telegraph* newspaper reported that samples from Ebola patients in West Africa had been exported without their consent and were being held in secret in laboratories across the world. The article reported that a laboratory was advertising virus samples online for a price quoted as being 170 times the price of gold (Freudenthal, 2019). Scientists and Ebola survivors in Africa accused the laboratories of biological asset stripping and requested their samples back for research. When questioned, the laboratory responded that they had shared the samples freely with other laboratories around the world and were also providing services such as sample extraction, purification, and characterization. Under European Union law at the time, the laboratory claimed to have intellectual property rights to offer it on the market at cost price. Ribeiro remarked that during outbreaks, researchers—particularly those in low- and middle-income countries (LMICs)—are often so busy supporting the response that they do not have the time or resources to engage in research. She added that most of those countries do not have facilities to store samples for future use; thus, they lose long-term access and control over samples.

Data Sharing in a Time of Transition

Data sharing has been in a time of transition since the 1990s, said Ribeiro. She traced the history of appropriation of resources without the fair sharing of benefit, which began with the adoption of the Agreement on Trade-Related Aspects of Intellectual Property Rights by the World Trade Organization in 1994. The trend toward appropriation was then driven by the genomics revolution in the 1990s through the 2000s, the development of technology for sequencing and bioprospecting, and the emergence of open-access databases. Many patents have been filed by companies in developed nations over resources and knowledge about how to apply resources coming from LMICs. However, these were later viewed as acts of biopiracy that became regulated under the Nagoya Protocol,[2] which was adopted in 2010 by the United Nations Environmental Programme at the Convention on Biological Diversity.

[2] More information on the Nagoya Protocol can be found at https://www.cbd.int/abs (accessed March 3, 2020).

The Nagoya Protocol established two principles: (1) the principle that countries have sovereign rights to decide and regulate how genetic resources coming from their countries are accessed and used, and (2) the principle of reciprocity, which gives countries the right to ask for a share of the benefits—monetary or otherwise—resulting from the use of such resources. She explained that this process led to a polarization and crisis of trust between providers and users of genetic resources. Because microorganisms and pathogens are included in the scope of the Nagoya Protocol, it changed the way that pathogen resources are shared globally, Ribeiro said. This paradigm change was driven by a series of shifts from:

- physical to digital environments;
- informal sharing to formal and regulated sharing;
- sharing at the national and regional scope to global sharing;
- sharing in isolated expert networks to sharing in more integrated systems involving multiple disciplines and sectors; and
- bilateral collaboration to complex multilevel cooperation.

Barriers to Sharing Pathogen Sequence Data

In association with the European COMPARE project, Ribeiro and colleagues identified barriers to sharing pathogen sequence data across domains, countries, sectors, and institutions (Ribeiro et al., 2018a). By plotting the barriers across the knowledge-valorization cycle for initiatives and innovations to tackle infectious diseases, they found that the barriers extended beyond different discourses, hampering early phases of pathogen discovery as well as the development of basic public health research and response measures. She highlighted several of the more complex barriers to frame her discussion of practical tools to improve collaboration and data sharing. Barriers related to research include publication priority, organizations' confidentiality, and insufficient compliance with ownership agreements. At the political and legal levels, barriers relate to countries' economies, international treaties, government permission, notification processes, ownership agreements, and political willingness among LMICs.

Practical Tools to Foster Collaboration and Enhance Sharing

Ribeiro suggested several practical tools for fostering collaboration and enhancing data sharing. Outbreak-related data need to be available before they are published, which would benefit from fostering a culture of rapid prepublished data sharing as an integral part of public health research. Funders and academic publishers should recognize the diversity of contributions and push for rapid publication through fast peer-review systems, preprint platforms, and alternative performance indicators for academic credit. Tools also need to be developed and implemented to improve coordination and establish trust, she suggested. To that end, database and collection curators should develop tools to build capacity, protect legitimate interests, and reinforce fair research collaborations.

For example, the COMPARE project has a database for sharing pathogen sequences and has established a pseudo-anonymized sharing platform in which it provides free and open access to analytical tools to help users interpret and use this data-building capacity. COMPARE has also experimented with different levels of access by providing private data hubs for users to share sensitive information with a selected group of stakeholders; after an agreed-upon duration, these data mandatorily go to the public domain. Ribeiro stated that the Global Initiative on Sharing All Influenza Data and the J. Craig Venter Institute have used access agreements to reinforce nonmonetary benefit sharing, in which users commit to engage in fair collaboration through co-authorships and acknowledgment of data providers.

Parallel legal databases and tracking systems have been useful for connecting shared materials and data with their legal documentations and conditions for use, she said. By providing transparency on rules and conditions, these can alleviate the demonstrative burden on users and help providers monitor access and benefit-sharing compliance. Blockchain-based systems have been used to link data, materials, and legal conditions, she added.

Developing Long-Term Policy and Legal Strategies

Ribeiro considered whether these practical tools are sufficient to solve the problems related to collaboration and data sharing to tackle microbial threats. Although these tools can alleviate some of the barriers, addressing the barriers' root causes—which are usually political and legal in nature—requires long-term policy and legal strategy recommendations. She offered three suggestions for establishing governance and legal preparedness.

Ribeiro's first suggestion was to define and clarify the scope of policies and regulations that govern data sharing. Discussions of global data sharing of pathogen resources often hinge on the scope and definitions of terms in the Nagoya Protocol (e.g., whether the term *genetic resources* includes only physical, biological materials or if the term also includes digital sequence data). She suggested that the focus of these discussions should shift from coverage issues to the effect of different modalities of implementation, given the importance of rapid access to sequence data in supporting outbreak research and response. The International Health Regulations also plays into these discussions. Although the framework determined that there is a need for rapid data sharing during public health emergencies of international concern (PHEICs),[3] it provides no specific guidance about which types of data should be shared, when they should be shared, or how they should be shared. The framework does not define the data-sharing obligations or establish a lower threshold for data sharing compared to a PHEIC. She suggested that obligations of rapid sharing should be established in advance.

Ribeiro's second suggestion was to coordinate epidemic research and development to organize the response and support rapid product development. She noted how the 2014 to 2016 Ebola outbreak in West Africa highlighted the importance of coordinated international response. Progress is being made under the World Health Organization (WHO) Blueprint Strategy, which is working with the Global Research Collaboration for Infectious Disease Preparedness and the Coalition for Epidemic Preparedness Innovations to connect affected countries with industry for rapid product development.

In the context of the One Health approach, she described the tripartite collaboration among WHO, the Food and Agriculture Organization of the United Nations, and the World Organisation for Animal Health to develop top-down guidance on the national and community implementation of One Health surveillance responses. However, she noted that this type of coordination mechanism takes time to be activated in practice because it is difficult to align these different organizations, as demonstrated by the issues faced during the MERS outbreak.

Developing harmonized and preestablished rules and conditions for data access, sharing, and use was Ribeiro's third suggestion. She explained that efficient data sharing requires harmonized systems based on simplified sharing agreements that have been established before times of crisis. The Network of International Exchange of Microbes under the Asian Consortium for the Conservation and Sustainable Use of Microbial Resources has a memorandum of understanding for noncommercial use of genetic resources that is an example of successful harmonization, she noted. Under this memorandum of understanding, all members waive their individual access and benefit-sharing conditions for sharing their resources for noncommercial use. Similarly, WHO's Pandemic Influenza Preparedness framework is multilateral and includes standard material transfer agreements to govern the sharing of materials for commercial use, which guarantees benefit sharing with industry (Ribeiro et al., 2018b).

---

[3] She defined a PHEIC as an occurrence or imminent threat of an illness or a health condition, caused by bioterrorism, epidemic or pandemic disease, or a novel and highly fatal infectious agent or biological toxin that poses a substantial risk of a significant number of human fatalities or incidents or permanent or long-term disability.

Promoting Outbreak-Related Data Sharing

Ribeiro remarked that despite the broad support and recognition of the need for data sharing to support outbreak research, data sharing during PHEICs remains limited. Technology is being developed at a pace that exceeds the development of governance mechanisms to implement those technologies and assess their social and economic effects, which has hampered efforts to apply these technologies in the most effective way. She suggested several areas of focus and investment to improve outbreak-related data sharing. Open-access databases are needed for outbreak research and response, but investment should also be channeled into developing collaborative platforms with curation strategies to support fair research collaborations and address the concerns of different stakeholders. Investment should also support efforts to build sharing systems during "peace time" that are substantiated by clear governance and legal mechanisms that can be rapidly activated and scaled up during times of crisis. Finally, she suggested that the focus should shift from the practice of bilateral negotiations toward global, harmonized, and preestablished systems for sharing pathogen resources that can support the timeliness and efficiency needed to support outbreak response.

ADDRESSING HEALTH CHALLENGES WITH BEHAVIORIAL INSIGHTS AND TOOLS

Fadi Makki explored strategies for applying insights from behavioral sciences to enhance acceptability and adoption of innovations across diverse social and cultural contexts. He described how behavioral insights can inform complementary tools to address health challenges using the example of a measles vaccination field experiment conducted in Lebanon.

Applying Evidence from Behavioral Science to Public Policy

Makki maintained that biases and other psychological determinants of health behavior need to be considered more thoroughly in order to apply behavioral insights to address health challenges, including microbial threats. Behavioral insights can offer complementary tools to health policy makers, he added. Evidence from behavioral science shows that decisions are not often deliberate or considered but automatic and influenced by context—that is, people do not make decisions in a straightforward way. He explained that among the psychological determinants involved in the processes of thinking, deciding, and taking action are misunderstandings, social pressure, information overload, overconfidence, procrastination, problems with willpower, forgetfulness, and inconvenience. One approach used to understand the biases and heuristics involved in decision making is dual system theory (Kahneman, 2003). Within this theory, system 1 thinking is faster and often used to make habitual decisions; this type of thinking is prone to error. System 2 thinking, which is used to make more complex decisions, has been described as a "lazy controller." He explained that the majority of thinking (approximately 90 percent) involves system 1, which he likened to cruise control.

Public policy often assumes that people tend to operate primarily with system 2 thinking to make decisions, said Makki. However, this assumption is being dispelled by a growing body of literature in psychology, economics, and public policy. The development of public policies has been dominated by tools that are based on rational assumptions that people are system 2 operators. These traditional tools fall along a spectrum with command-and-control approaches on one end, rewards and incentives on the other, and the basic provision of information in the middle. He explained that command-and-control approaches rely on sanctions and penalties, which do not always work, while the use of rewards and incentives is not a sustainable approach.

The basic provision of information relies on assumptions that people have greater cognitive processing power than they actually do. However, policy makers can avail themselves of complementary tools anchored in behavioral insights that can be helpful, said Makki. For instance, the concept of "nudging" is a behavioral insight tool that refers to "any aspect of choice architecture that alters people's behavior in a predictable way without forbidding any options or significantly changing their economic incentives" (Thaler and Sunstein, 2009). He suggested that applying these types of behavioral insights from multidisciplinary research in fields such as economics, psychology, sociology, cognitive science, and neuroscience is relevant to all policy areas and can be used to inform better understanding about how humans behave.

Using Behavioral Insights to Address Health Challenges: Example from Lebanon

Behavioral insights can be used to address health challenges by exploring the behavior of individual patients and their families. Makki explained that behavioral bottlenecks exist at every level of the behavioral change pathway—prevention, early detection, and treatment—and are encountered by every stakeholder in the value change. He explained that these bottlenecks can be addressed through a two-step process. The first step is to review biases through a behavioral lens by evaluating psychological determinants. The second step is to use experiments to test approaches to changing behavior, ideally with randomized controlled trials.

To illustrate this process, Makki described a randomized controlled trial conducted in Lebanon to increase uptake of the measles vaccine during an outbreak. As part of the study, they evaluated the challenges and biases that affect individuals' decisions about vaccination and developed solutions to address some of these challenges and biases to shape people's behavior, he said. Figure 4-1 provides a list of psychological biases and bottlenecks they identified during this process. For instance, present bias makes the benefits of vaccination less salient or immediately available, while the costs, side effects, pain, effort, and inconvenience of vaccination are immediate. Optimism bias can cause parents to underestimate the consequences of their child contracting a viral disease. He noted that the status quo bias was especially relevant for parents who were used to receiving vaccination services at school or at their doorstep.

Other challenges identified during the trial included neglect, forgetfulness, previous bad experiences with primary health care, lack of awareness, and perceptions of low quality. Many of these challenges and biases have behavioral roots that can be countered by different types of interventions. Makki and colleagues created the SHAPE DIFFERENCE strategy to develop and test various interventions that are informed by behavioral insight tools (see Figure 4-2). For example, planning prompts ask beneficiaries to write down or choose the day and time they intend to act on something, such as having their children vaccinated. Making a public commitment, receiving reminders, and social norms can also have an effect on behavior. He noted that "default" is among the most powerful nudges. This can be used by defaulting beneficiaries into prescheduled time slots with an opportunity to

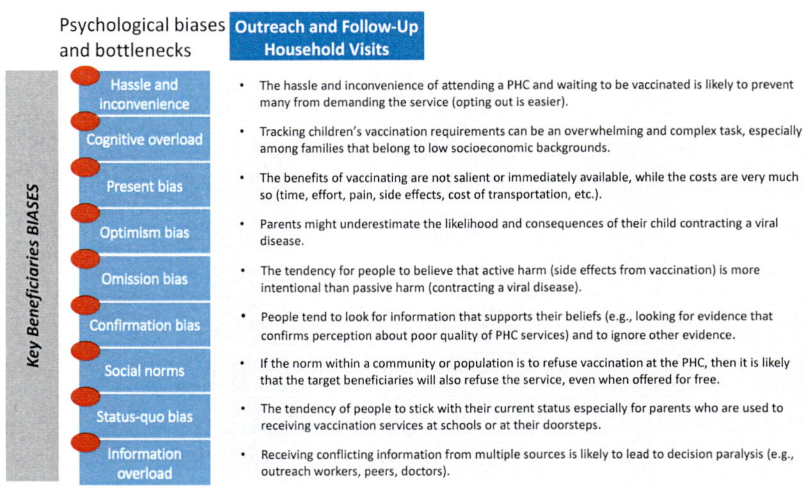

FIGURE 4-1 Behavioral insights from Nudge Lebanon randomized controlled trials.
NOTE: PHC = primary health care.
SOURCES: Makki presentation, December 4, 2019; B4Development and Nudge Lebanon team analysis.

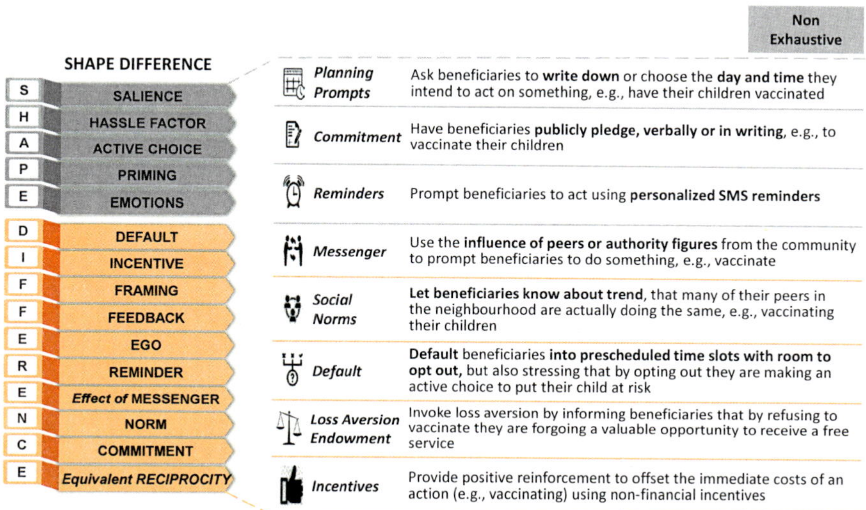

FIGURE 4-2 Behavioral insight tools.
SOURCES: Makki presentation, December 4, 2019; B4Development and Nudge Lebanon team analysis.

opt out, while also emphasizing that opting out is making an active choice to put the child at risk.

Findings and Lessons Learned from the Measles Vaccination Field Experiment

To evaluate the benefits of SHAPE DIFFERENCE behavioral insights, Makki and colleagues developed a test calendar, comprising five nudges and behavioral tools; this calendar was used in 6,160 households across three areas of Lebanon, Makki explained. The calendar was designed to counter the negative influences of peers, the discontent from receiving the same services as refugees, neglect, intention–action gap, forgetfulness, lack of trust in the quality of vaccines at the primary health center, and the lack of awareness that vaccination is free. For example, based on the social norms insight, the calendar informs beneficiaries that more than 90,000 children have already been vaccinated free of charge. The calendar uses social endorsement and commitment by informing beneficiaries that their neighbors are protecting their children by vaccinating them and asking beneficiaries to check a box promising to vaccinate their own children. The calendar again uses the commitment insight by asking beneficiaries to put a nonbinding sticker on the calendar marking the day they will bring their children to be vaccinated. The intention of this aspect of the implementation is to bridge the intention–action gap by prompting beneficiaries to mark a day on the calendar.

Finally, the calendar uses the effect of messenger insight by displaying the seal of the Ministry of Health. This insight was used to address the fact that many people thought the vaccinations delivered at primary health centers were of low quality. Use of the calendar during this trial led to a 50 percent increase in the likelihood of vaccinating relative to the control group that did not receive the calendar, Makki reported. The probability of a household vaccinating at least one child was 6.8 percentage points greater among the treatment group households (20.3 percent) than the control group households (13.5 percent). In terms of vaccination uptake by visit type, uptake was 5.7 percentage points greater among the treatment group than the control group via outreach and 9.3 percentage points greater among the treatment group versus the control group via follow-up.

Makki provided an overview of lessons learned from the experiment. The first was that applying the same solution to different populations will produce different results. Non-Lebanese beneficiaries were more likely to trust that the vaccines offered by primary health centers were truly free and were 4.4 percentage points more likely to vaccinate their children than Lebanese households. It is also necessary to develop a proper understanding of the target population and the behavioral challenges deterring them from acting on their intentions. Using the behavior change tools in the calendar, Makki and colleagues identified common recurring problems among their participants. However, he cautioned that the use of behavioral insights does not represent a perfect solution to structural problems, but rather complements conventional procedures.

In the case of the measles vaccination experiment, the majority of households involved in the experiment remained unvaccinated; although the treatment led to measurable improvement, it did not solve the problem of undervaccination. Lastly, he observed that offering the same message repeatedly did not necessarily lead to higher uptake. Multiple outreach visits can increase uptake but only if coupled with new offerings. In this case, households receiving the calendar during a follow-up visit were 9.3 percentage points more likely to vaccinate compared to those that did not.

Apply Behavioral Insights to Other Stakeholders to Counter Microbial Threats

Makki explored the need to focus on other stakeholders when applying behavioral insights to the area of microbial threats. Focusing exclusively on individual behavior does not account for the behavior of other stakeholders in the value chain, such as industry, policy makers, and health care providers.

Behavioral insight tools can also be used to nudge these other stakeholders into a course of action. To illustrate the application of these insights to addressing antimicrobial resistance, he described how behavioral insights can be used to counter the overprescription of antibiotics. Antibiotic resistance is a key threat to global health, with many infections becoming more resistant to treatment as antibiotics become less effective; health care systems also face mounting costs as a result of antibiotic misuse and overuse.

He highlighted several behavioral insight tools that can be used to help address this issue. Social norms are commonly used to discourage overprescription of antibiotics by comparing physicians' rates of prescription. For example, an intervention in the United Kingdom sends personalized letters to the most overprescribing physicians to inform them that 80 percent of doctors prescribe fewer antibiotics. These letters were sent by the UK Chief Medical Officer, using the effect of messenger, another behavioral insight tool. These letters were associated with a significant drop in the prescription of antibiotics, he said (Hallsworth et al., 2016).

To use the commitment tool, another intervention hung poster-sized letters in exam rooms for 3 months that included photographs and signatures of doctors who committed not to prescribe antibiotics unnecessarily. The intervention group decreased their antibiotic prescribing rates by 9.1 percent, while the control group's prescribing rate increased by 9.2 percent (Meeker et al., 2014). Hand hygiene is another area in which behavioral insights can be used to counter hospital-acquired infections and antimicrobial resistance, he added.

Advancing the Application of Behavioral Insights

Makki concluded with a set of takeaway messages and potential avenues for applying behavioral insights to counter antimicrobial resistance. Expectations must be managed, he said. The power of behavioral insights has become increasingly recognized in recent years, but behavioral insights are not a panacea. In some cases, more traditional regulation- or incentive-based tools will still be needed. Behavioral insights should be treated as complementary tools, rather than strict alternatives. He noted that context matters—what works in one place will not necessarily work in another place, which underscores the need to test tools and experiment using rigorous evaluation methods.

Scaling up the use of behavioral sciences in public policy and health policy through capacity building across all stakeholders in the health care value chain will allow for more opportunity for cocreation, he suggested. Behavioral insights courses are being taught to new civil service graduates; health care providers would benefit from being taught about them as well. He added that social norms are a powerful tool, but dynamic social norms are even better. Dynamic social norms inform beneficiaries that the norm is trending upward, which has a larger effect in terms of updating peoples' beliefs and countering fake news. Makki and colleagues are working to create a game to inoculate people against fake news related to vaccines, for example.

DISCUSSION

Eva Harris opened the discussion by reflecting on each of the presentations. She remarked that Osewe illustrated the benefits of creating a straightforward platform to support health workers on the ground in LMICs, as well as providing population-wide analytics; he also underscored the challenge of how to foster local-level innovation in the face of competition from innovations developed by larger international organizations that may not be suited to local needs. She highlighted Bird's focus on the local community being a key stakeholder in the uptake of epidemic response activities, as evidenced by the Ebola outbreak, and on the need to understand and adapt to local cultural contexts. Harris commented that Ribeiro's presentation showed why practical tools to foster collaborations need to be put in place ahead of, during, and after the public health emergencies. Makki's presentation elucidated how behavioral tools can be experimentally applied to change behaviors, said Harris, which offers a potential strategy for dealing with health issues such as loss of confidence in vaccines in a culturally respectful way.

Matthew Zahn, medical director, Division of Epidemiology and Assessment, Orange County Health Care Agency, asked if data sharing has actually improved over the past decade. Ribeiro responded that the question reveals a common sentiment across researchers in this area that these issues are too complex to resolve. Although there have been successful systems at a small scale or tackling specific resources, much progress remains to be made toward an overarching solution. However, she noted progress over the past decade in how data are shared, as evidenced by gene banks, global networks, and discussions under way at WHO, at the Convention on Biological Diversity, and in regional networks such as the European Commission. Harris pointed out that discussions at the organizational level may not include in-country interaction. Ribeiro replied that these discussions are centered at a political level; more engagement is needed with researchers who share data, use data, and coordinate the response.

Maurizio Vecchione, executive vice president of Global Good and Research, Intellectual Ventures, asked Bird to expand on the communication strategies used to share public health information about the Bombali and Marburg viruses with local communities as well as internationally. Bird replied that decisions about how to handle this type of information are complicated and political, because they are determined by the situation and setting. If a virus is found that is closely related to known pathogens, that information must be disseminated, which has ramifications for people on the ground.

In a small country like Sierra Leone, it is easier to access the president or the minister of health than in a country like Tanzania, he added. When they found the Bombali virus, it was challenging to convince governments of countries to take the threat seriously and develop a rational response, which he attributed in part to the psychological ramifications of the recent Ebola outbreak. Over a period of a few weeks, however, they were able to work with government colleagues (including the highest-level officials) to develop the communication materials to deliver to communities. He noted this strategy was in keeping with the ethos of the PREDICT project of making a country's priorities superordinate to a program's priorities. This process of communication and activating a response is more immediate and straightforward for a virus like Marburg, which is a known human pathogen, noted Bird.

In contrast, after the discovery of the Bombali virus they encountered some resistance from the academic community, despite concrete laboratory confirmation of the existence of the virus, about whether to tell the public immediately or to wait for a peer-review process to publish a paper. With the government's support they decided to go ahead and release information in the country, which included visits to local communities. He commented that the community level should not be overlooked in discussions about data sharing, particularly in the context of sharing information about high-consequence pathogens at the village level. For instance, his group has developed a "bat book" to inform people in their local language about how to co-exist safely with bats, who are good for the environment but sometimes carry viruses or pathogens that harm humans.

George Haringhuizen, coordinating advisor and senior legal counsel, Dutch National Institute for Public Health and the Environment, commented that his group has convened many workshops with hundreds of scientists, asking what they would do if they were to discover a new pathogen, in terms of reporting to the government or going for publication. He said that more than half of those scientists said they would go immediately for publication to disseminate the information, while the remainder said governments should be informed so they can manage the possible outbreak. Haringhuizen commented that the approach described by Bird showed how the community can be engaged in research and development of an outbreak response.

Greg Armstrong said that Bird made a good case for having a process in place to deal with the discovery of previously unknown viruses not yet found in humans. He asked how researchers might prepare in advance for transmitting these types of results. Bird responded that it should be part of the scientific culture to determine in advance how to deal with the discovery of an infectious pathogen. He pointed out that such discoveries are like a microcosm of an outbreak in terms of the urgency to plan, to find partners, and to identify key players in the country—these steps can be taken in advance of initiating a research project. He described Ebola as the acid test of a worst-case pathogen discovery effort because "Fearbola is bigger than Ebola." To mitigate these issues, he suggested working from the outset of a project with government colleagues at all levels to ensure they understand the potential ramifications for the community, country, and region, including trade implications. For example, veterinary diseases can have substantial regulatory and economic implications. He suggested that to err on the side of caution, any new pathogen should be considered a potentially robust human pathogen until proven otherwise.

Rafael Obregón asked about how to integrate behavioral tools into disease outbreak response, because many community engagement interventions are setting specific and not easily replicable. Makki responded that context does matter and that experiments cannot be replicated exactly, but lessons can be gleaned from previous work when implementing in a new setting in order to further refine and improve the experiment. He suggested that capacity building and integrating behavior science at every step could help support efforts to scale up interventions more broadly. This effort would also benefit from educating more stakeholders—including policy makers, health care providers, and nongovernmental organizations (NGOs)—about the advantages of applying behavioral science and incorporating it into their work.

Harris asked Osewe about barriers they encountered as a local NGO trying to bring their innovation into practical use in the clinics and beyond. Osewe responded that in his experience, innovation is about creating value in addressing the real challenges that people are facing on the ground. Their platform was more readily accepted by end users because they had involved them in designing the concept, technology, and infrastructure. He added that partnership is also critical for scaling up. He suggested that the first phase of rolling out an innovation should involve engaging with decision makers, hospital and clinic managers, and volunteers to obtain buy-in and promote scalability.

Jonathan Towner asked about how to manage sample sharing for pathogens such as Ebola, which have biosecurity and safety concerns. He suggested that bilateral agreements might be an efficient way to get samples out of insecure areas. Ribeiro responded that infectious diseases do not respect boundaries and require global collaboration for the response, which necessitates continued international support for storing samples and developing countermeasures. She suggested moving forward initially by building local capacity to store and analyze samples. In terms of global sharing, she noted that bilateral negotiations are complicated, especially when they occur in times of crisis. Ideally, harmonized international agreements would be developed at the global level with conditions that are equal for every country, she said.

Reflections on Day 1 of the Workshop

Kent Kester, vice president and head, translational science and biomarkers, Sanofi Pasteur, closed the first day of the workshop by highlighting what he considered to be a set of recurring issues discussed by various speakers:

- The metrics for success for new discoveries and approaches used in academia are often discordant with translational success in terms of deployment, implementation, or changes in policy and practice that make a difference in people's lives.
- Substantial gaps remain in implementation and sustainability. Strong pilot projects and promising developments in vaccines and therapeutics often stall because they do not have the activation energy to be implemented sustainably at large scale, owing to a host of barriers that are difficult to overcome.
- Better strategies are needed to understand, build trust, and foster engagement with communities in the realms of research, outbreak response, and delivery of new technological approaches.
- Demonstrating value across health, financial, and social dimensions can help to accelerate the implementation of innovative projects.
- Innovative approaches should strive to be transversal, with connectivity across a range of problem areas; for example, mobile health apps could be designed to manage a range of diseases instead of just one.
- Data sharing is complicated by a host of factors—from national sovereignty to intellectual property to monetization of data—but these issues must be resolved, because infectious diseases do not respect country boundaries.
- Behavioral sciences can offer insights into how to engage with stakeholders and communities to facilitate the uptake of innovations in supportive rather than directive ways.

5

Systems Approaches to Spur Innovations in Tackling Antimicrobial Resistance

The third session of the workshop focused on antimicrobial resistance (AMR) and examined systematic approaches to stimulate innovations in AMR. Speakers and discussants explored the elements of policy, regulatory, market, and funding environments that could foster innovation in the field to address AMR; novel strategies to facilitate the mitigation of the burden of AMR; and promising avenues for coordination across systems to advance innovation in AMR. The session was moderated by Cristina Cassetti, deputy division director, Division of Microbial and Infectious Diseases, National Institute of Allergy and Infectious Diseases. Christine Kreuder Johnson, professor of epidemiology and ecosystem health, University of California, Davis, shared lessons from the One Health approach used in Kathmandu, Nepal, to enhance animal and human surveillance systems to bolster innovation in AMR.

Wes Kim, senior officer, Antibiotic Resistance Project, The Pew Charitable Trusts, discussed the development and implementation of the Shared Platform for Antibiotic Research and Knowledge (SPARK) platform, which is spurring antibiotic discovery through data sharing. Daniel Berman, lead, Longitude Prize, shared how Nesta is incentivizing novel diagnostic tests to counter antibiotic resistance with the Longitude Prize. Jyoti Joshi, head of the South Asia Center for Disease Dynamics, Economics & Policy (CDDEP), discussed approaches to strengthening health systems in order to overcome market and regulatory barriers to innovation in AMR.

APPLYING LESSONS FROM ONE HEALTH SURVEILLANCE TO TACKLE ANTIMICROBIAL RESISTANCE

Christine Kreuder Johnson explored how using a One Health approach to enhance animal and human surveillance systems can bolster innovation in AMR. She described the typical surveillance design that was used across 27 countries in the U.S. Agency for International Development's (USAID's) PREDICT project, which engaged with countries to bolster animal and human surveillance within communities, and she provided a case presentation of this design that was implemented in a temporary settlement in Kathmandu, Nepal.

One Health Surveillance in Kathmandu, Nepal

The PREDICT program developed an innovative approach informed by One Health called triangulation to conduct coordinated animal and human surveillance to identify zoonotic pathogens at high-risk animal–human interfaces, said Johnson. The approach involves (1) the concurrent sampling of people, livestock, and wildlife within their shared habitat at points of epidemiological contact; and (2) the incorporation of behavioral and social science through detailed questionnaires and surveys to investigate behavioral and social factors and inform risk mitigation and interventions. Central to the PREDICT project was engaging with communities to perform zoonotic disease surveillance within the community as a discrete epidemiological unit.

Johnson presented Figure 5-1, which depicts the temporary settlement community in Kathmandu where PREDICT's surveillance model was used. While the PREDICT team was looking for viral threats in this community, they decided to take advantage of the opportunity to look for AMR as well. To pilot this innovation, they sampled across sectors using a One Health surveillance approach for 1 week to get a "snapshot" of AMR in the community.[1] They engaged households in study enrollment and sampled several members of each household, sampled animals that were being reared, sampled wildlife active around homes or in nearby crops, and sampled the water from the nearby river. All work was conducted using appropriate biosafety practices for sampling. She added that they also looked for avian influenza in the community, because significant close contact between animals and humans in this setting presented many opportunities for sharing viral pathogens and AMR. The Center for Molecular Dynamics, a team fostering and implementing surveillance in Nepal, took on this work. This

[1] Johnson noted that PREDICT also engaged with the local health care facility to conduct syndromic surveillance for viral threats, but microbial resistance was surveilled through only the community.

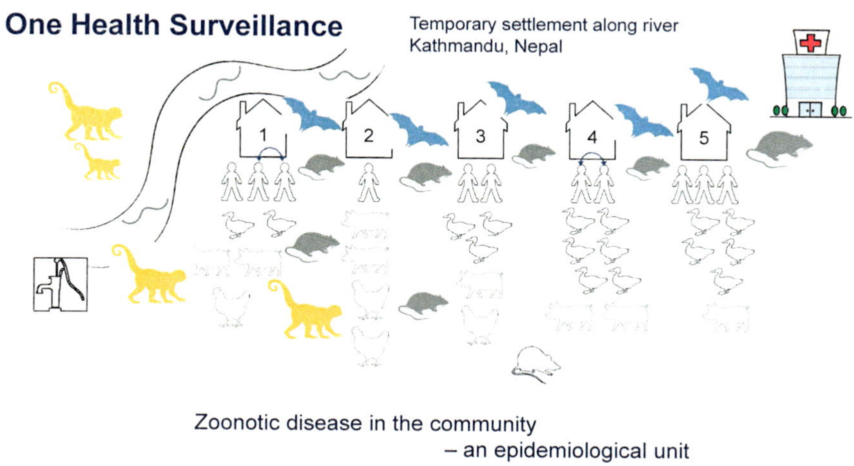

FIGURE 5-1 Zoonotic disease in the community—an epidemiological unit.
SOURCES: Johnson presentation, December 5, 2019; information from USAID.

team set up a laboratory in a house in this settlement and implemented the biosafety measures necessary to sample wildlife and other species.

Outcomes of One Health Surveillance

Johnson provided an overview of the outcomes of PREDICT's One Health Surveillance in the community in Kathmandu. The team screened a subset of samples for 88 AMR genes using quantitative polymerase chain reaction, and preliminary findings revealed that 69 of 88 AMR genes were detected in the community. Among the humans sampled, some predictive factors were identified. The burden of resistance increased with age, but having a dedicated location for trash, animal waste, and human waste each decreased the risk. Keeping animals increased the risk, with the highest burden of resistance found in households that kept swine. Households with animals had an average of 11.4 resistance genes, while those without animals had an average of 5.0 resistance genes. The fecal samples from humans, ducks, and chickens revealed a tremendous amount of sharing of AMR genes, she noted, and most humans in the community had most of the circulating AMR genes. She suggested that this was likely attributable to the close contact among animals and humans in the community.

Johnson explained that they developed a novel way to visualize the community sharing of AMR genes by pairing samples from animal, human, and water sources, as shown in Figure 5-2. Wildlife had the fewest AMR genes overall, and their AMR genes had less in common with those in humans and

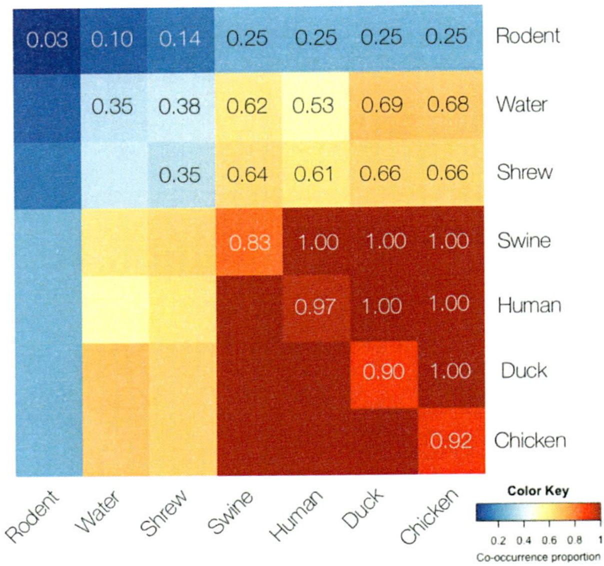

FIGURE 5-2 Antimicrobial resistance gene co-occurrence among humans, animals, and environment in a community context in Kathmandu, Nepal.
SOURCES: Johnson presentation, December 5, 2019; information from USAID.

livestock. Rodents had very little resistance but shrews that were trapped in people's homes had greater levels of resistance. Swine, humans, ducks, and chickens had the highest levels of resistance overall. Among humans, ducks, and swine, every sample tested had at least one shared AMR gene. The PREDICT team also compared oral versus fecal sample types, she said. AMR genes were more similar in chicken and duck oral samples, while chicken, duck, and human fecal samples were the most similar. Although AMR was not found in the drinking water, it was found in water along the river.

Implications of AMR in the Environment

The preliminary findings from surveillance in the community in Kathmandu motivated hypotheses related to opportunities for transmission in the type of close-knit communities where there are dense livestock holdings and human communities, Johnson said. Even though the researchers did not find high prevalence in these particular samples, this setting had high potential for AMR in wildlife and possibly in other reservoirs such as waters, soil, and crops. Wildlife are underrecognized in terms of AMR, noted Johnson. Even minor amounts of AMR in wildlife can be an issue when methods for control and decreasing resistance begin to be implemented through antimicrobial use, continued Johnson. If AMR genes are shared with wildlife through shared habitats with people, it could cause a problem for ongoing control. For instance, AMR in bats could be a potential threat to food safety, because they tend to live in dense areas and congregate in settings close to humans; their guano is also harvested and spread on crops as fertilizer. She highlighted this as an example of how resistance in wildlife—even among a species that is not typically thought of as sharing a habitat with humans—can spill back into at-risk human populations. This illustrates how much room there is for innovation in global surveillance for AMR, she said.

Challenges and Opportunities in Global Surveillance of Antimicrobial Resistance

Johnson touched on challenges and opportunities in global surveillance for AMR. Johnson said that the challenges to AMR surveillance are similar to the challenges faced for zoonotic disease surveillance in general. For instance, global disparities proliferate; low- and middle-income countries (LMICs) tend to have the greatest burdens of AMR but the most limited resources to improve surveillance. Gaps in the evidence base remain large, she added. As with zoonotic diseases, evidence is needed to fill these gaps to inform transmission-based interventions for disease control as the foundation for infectious disease control everywhere. She suggested that research could focus on prioritization of high-risk environments, movement of AMR from health care facilities to livestock holdings and the community, the importance of cross-species transmission, and directionality of transmission.

In a recent study, researchers used metagenomic analysis of untreated sewage to characterize the bacterial resistome across 60 different countries (Hendriksen et al., 2019). They found a strong correlation between abundance of AMR, sanitation, and health indices. These findings echo the findings of PREDICT in Kathmandu on a much broader scale, Johnson added.

Johnson highlighted USAID's vision of tackling pandemic threats and training One Health workforces as a defining moment for countering microbial threats: there are opportunities for success in having human health and animal health coordinated in the field, being sampled and tested together. However, government engagement will be needed to facilitate policy change, and community engagement will be needed to facilitate behavior change. Supportive policies to tackle AMR could help to coordinate surveillance, convene data streams, and harmonize reporting frameworks to include humans, animals, and the environment. PREDICT has done this to standardize reporting across humans and animals.

Johnson noted that the World Health Organization (WHO) is also doing this for humans, but including animal and environmental data in WHO reporting going forward would be key in standardizing reporting frameworks.

USAID's vision of engaging scientific colleagues around the world in the One Health strategy could support global AMR efforts, she suggested. The One Health workforce consists of more than 6,200 people working in more than 60 laboratories in 30 countries; they have already sampled more than 145,000 animals and humans as part of the PREDICT project, helping to minimize the spillover of zoonotic disease threats from animals into human populations (Cima, 2020). They have detected more than 1,100 unique viruses, including zoonotic diseases of public health concern, such as Bombali Ebola virus, Zaire Ebola virus, Marburg virus, and MERS- and SARS-like coronaviruses[2] (Cima, 2020). She emphasized the need to have people working in the field in advance of outbreaks who have the skills for ethical sampling of both humans and animals. The PREDICT project in Kathmandu demonstrated that the PREDICT strategy could be applied to AMR and yield informative findings, she noted.

SPARKING ANTIBIOTIC DISCOVERY THROUGH DATA SHARING AND SCIENTIFIC COLLABORATION

Wes Kim presented on an innovative avenue for data sharing and scientific collaboration to spur antibiotic discovery. SPARK is an online data discovery tool being provided to the Bio-X discovery community to help catalyze the discovery and development of new antibiotics.

Pipeline Analysis of Antibiotic Candidates in Development

Pew's recent pipeline analysis demonstrated continued insufficient candidates in development, said Kim. For the past 5 years, Pew has been tracking the global pipeline for clinical candidates, including both small molecules and "nontraditionals," which tend to be biologics, but Kim focused on the small molecules. As of Pew's last report, there were 37 small molecules in clinical development, 4 in new drug application review, and 1 that had received a complete response. He noted that year after year, the total number of candidates in clinical development has been steady—ranging between the upper 30s and lower 40s—but most of those candidates will never be approved, and the 42 current candidates will decline sharply as they go through clinical development. Of the 42 current candidates, 17 target the gram-negative bacteria among the ESKAPE (*Enterococcus faecium, Staphylococcus aureus, Klebsiella pneumoniae, Acinetobacter baumannii, Pseudomonas aeruginosa,* and *Enterobacter species*) pathogens.

The ESKAPE pathogens are considered superbugs because of their higher affinity for developing resistance, so these 17 candidates could potentially fulfill an unmet public health need (The Pew Charitable Trusts,

[2] MERS is Middle East respiratory syndrome and SARS is severe acute respiratory syndrome.

2019a). Pew also tracks the novelty of drug candidates, because clinicians and infectious disease doctors need drugs that provide either novel scaffolds or novel mechanisms of action that potentially help delay the development of resistance. Pew's evaluation found that only 1 of the 17 candidates in the clinical pipeline that target gram-negative ESKAPE pathogens represents a novel class candidate. Unfortunately, that candidate has since been discontinued because of toxicity issues. Kim said that although the three approvals that occurred in 2019 are cause for optimism, it is important to stay adamant in pushing for the development of new antibiotics.

Development of the Shared Platform for Antibiotic Research and Knowledge

Kim traced the development of Pew's SPARK tool. Between 2014 and 2015, Pew convened leaders in the field of antibiotics discovery to catalyze the development of antibiotics by creating a Scientific Roadmap for Antibiotic Discovery (Talkington et al., 2016). They considered the scientific gaps that are contributing to the lack of novel discoveries and new antibiotics and identified three overarching priorities: guidelines for drug discovery, new starting material and chemical scaffold, and a platform for knowledge exchange. New starting material might include three to five physical and chemical properties of small molecules that allow them to penetrate and remain in the pathogens. A knowledge-sharing platform is needed to ensure that work does not just sit on the shelf.

The leaders also expressed concern about market instability for the development of new antibiotics. Together, these three priorities underscored the need for a platform for collaborating and sharing results from studies to answer gram-negative efflux and permeation questions and to collate lessons learned to minimize unnecessary redundancy in future research endeavors. Kim explained that based on those three priorities, Pew designed and launched the SPARK platform. Box 5-1 provides more details about SPARK. The SPARK database has already received contributions from industry, including Novartis and Achaogen (The Pew Charitable Trusts, 2018, 2019b,c), and they are currently in discussions with other pharmaceutical and biotechnology companies that are interested in sharing data. SPARK also collects data from academic nonprofit organizations who screen compounds for their contractor; once those data are released, they are added to SPARK. The platform was launched in 2018 and currently has more than 600 registrants.

Challenges to Implementing a Data-Sharing Platform

Kim remarked that operationalizing SPARK was challenging in several respects. He shared some of the challenges that Pew encountered and

BOX 5-1
Shared Platform for Antibiotic Research and Knowledge (SPARK)

The Pew Charitable Trusts developed the Shared Platform for Antibiotic Research and Knowledge (SPARK) as an upstream, interactive, publicly available online discovery tool with a strong focus on the early stages of discovery, small molecules, and gram-negative pathogens. Nontraditionals, gram-positive pathogens, clinical human data, and animal data are outside the scope of SPARK. The platform is narrowly focused on early-stage discovery to address the gap highlighted by the scientific community. SPARK is free to use; anyone can sign up and get credentials to access the data on the platform. The platform is constantly expanding its compound libraries with associated physiochemical properties and assay data.

The platform offers curated data from diverse sources based on assay type, rather than data source; it also provides computational modeling and trend analyses to assess cellular entry and target inhibition. The platform is not a mere repository for depositing data. SPARK discovery experts, who have 30–40 years of expertise, work behind the scenes to process the collected data; they annotate assay condition in order to allow each lab to do an apples-to-apples comparison between assays. This is valuable because each lab tweaks its own assays, which can make it difficult to directly compare assays. SPARK also offers computational modeling and other analysis tools that allow registrants to access and use data in accordance with their needs.

SOURCE: Kim presentation, December 5, 2019.

explained how they are working to mitigate those challenges. The implementation of SPARK raised concerns about intellectual property. He noted that Pew does not expect lead assets to be shared; rather, they hope that stakeholders will consider sharing inactive programs or completed programs that are sitting on the shelf. For instance, one company that has patented compound structures but has not released the biological activity data was comfortable sharing chemical structure data. Pew is working to further mitigate challenges related to intellectual property concerns and make organizations comfortable sharing their data, he added.

The implementation of SPARK also encountered challenges because of disparate formats and sources of data, said Kim. For example, a gap in the field of antibiotics discovery is the development of an assay to measure the extent to which a compound gets into a pathogen, where it gets in, and where it accumulates. Researchers currently use a range of different methodologies for this work, which makes it difficult to compare data across laboratories. SPARK is working with their discovery experts to collate these data by identifying certain assays that provide sufficient data and congruence across multiple laboratories. That will allow SPARK to provide collated, curated data to the community and thus enable the community to work on new ways to address antibiotic permeation and accumulation.

Finally, Kim highlighted the challenge of growing critical mass and ensuring sustained usefulness for SPARK. They are creating strategies to build awareness and maintain interest in the platform. For example, they announce data donations periodically and are developing an ambassador program of researchers who use SPARK regularly. These ambassadors are working in the field, speaking at conferences, publishing, and publicly talking about how they use SPARK in their own research. Kim said that ultimately, SPARK is not for Pew—it was designed by scientists for scientists. Their aim is to grow the database and provide data that will be used for in vitro data analysis, which will then be channeled back into SPARK to facilitate the discovery of novel antibiotics.

INCENTIVIZING NOVEL DIAGNOSTIC TESTS TO COUNTER ANTIBIOTIC RESISTANCE

Daniel Berman presented on incentivizing novel diagnostic tests to counter AMR. His organization, Nesta, is an innovation foundation with a focus on implementation rather than the act of innovating; they seek out projects that bring together technology and innovation to address social objectives. The mission of Nesta Challenges is to stimulate and speed up problem-solving activity on the most difficult challenges society faces, especially ones that are being overlooked. Nesta Challenges uses innovation competitions to excite and engage the broadest community of problem solvers and create solutions that are high quality, sustainable, and impactful. Unlike traditional grants or other methodologies, Nesta has people compete with each other against a defined objective.[3]

Nesta's Longitude Prize

Berman described one of Nesta Challenges's initiatives, the Longitude Prize. It is a £10 million prize fund with an £8 million prize payout to one winner that will reward a transformative, rapid, accurate, and affordable point-of-care diagnostic test that can significantly reduce antibiotic misuse or overuse, anywhere in the world. The first applicant to "pass the post" wins the entire prize. To register for the prize, applicants must prove their vision matches the vision of the Longitude Prize project. He explained that

[3] More information about the Nesta Challenges methodology is available from https://challenges.org/impact/reports/nesta-challenges-practice-guide-2019 (accessed February 6, 2020).

the second step, registering to win, is much more difficult—only 20 applicants had registered to win the prize as of December 2019. To win the prize, competitors must meet the following eight specific criteria with a rapid, point-of-care diagnostic test that reduces inappropriate antibiotic prescribing and is accurate, affordable, and impactful globally:

1. Needed: The test must improve the antibiotic treatment decisions related to this globally occurring problem.
2. Accurate: The test must eliminate harmful treatment decisions and give confidence to the user.
3. Affordable: The test must be affordable for purchase and use everywhere that it is needed.
4. Rapid: The test must deliver a result in less than 30 minutes from sample collection.
5. Easy to use: The test can be used and interpreted anywhere in the world without advanced medical resources.[4]
6. Scalable: It is an original idea with a plan for full-scale manufacture and distribution.
7. Safe: The benefits of using the test far outweigh any risks associated with it.
8. Connected: The test has built-in data recording and transmission capability.

By definition, these types of prizes are designed to be difficult challenges, Berman remarked. Typically, test designers would make trade-offs among these criteria, but the Longitude Prize requires all eight criteria to be met. In addition to the eight criteria, the test should also be environmentally stable and easily carried, and it should not require a cold chain, household electricity, or a laboratory technician to deliver results. In terms of accuracy, the prize rules do not specify a necessary degree of specificity or sensitivity, because those factors are context specific, but the winning test must be accurate enough to be clinically useful.

Overview of the Ongoing Competition

Berman said that as of December 2019, 55 teams were in the competition, including start-up companies, academic groups, and midsized diagnostic companies.[5] The teams come from Australia, Belgium, Canada, France, India,

[4] Berman noted that it must truly be a point-of-care test; for example, the commonly used Cepheid test would not be considered a point-of-care test.

[5] More information on competing teams can be found at https://longitudeprize.org/teams (accessed March 3, 2020).

Israel, Malaysia, the Netherlands, Sweden, Turkey, and the United Kingdom. Teams are working on a range of different test types, including bacterial versus viral differentiation, pathogen identification, antibiotic susceptibility testing, urinary tract infections, and tests for blood infections such as sepsis. Novel projects involving microfluidics, lateral flow, biosensor/biowire, and polymerase chain reaction are some of the technologies being deployed, he said, with many teams are utilizing multiple technologies. Some teams competing for the prize have developed projects that are quite novel, he added.

Berman said that the tests that are being developed for the Longitude Prize fall into two categories: (1) tests that are designed for the U.S. and European markets that are finding venture capital and national government support, and (2) tests that are designed for LMICs that are struggling to find financing, investment, and joint-venture-type collaborations. He pointed out that there are many tests in the latter category that would have significant impact if successful, but many of these tests are stalled in development owing to lack of investment.

Teams are required to self-fund for the most part, although they are also supported through grants, investment funding, and technical support. Nesta estimates that teams will need at least £30 million to bring a diagnostic test to market. Berman pointed out that diagnostics do not have the same quick uptake once they are brought to market, which is an additional challenge. He reported that 29 teams were awarded Discovery Awards of £25,000, 3 Longitude Prize teams were awarded boost grants of up to £100,000 by the Biotechnology Industry Research Assistance Council, and three initial investments will be made from a £3 million impact investment fund established by an anonymous donor. Some of the teams from India and the United Kingdom have been hosted by accelerators or incubators. He added that to foster collaboration and provide access to experts, Nesta Challenges convenes workshops on commercial plans, intellectual property, and regulatory filing.

Opportunities to Improve the Longitude Prize

Berman discussed some aspects of the Longitude Prize that, in hindsight, Nesta would do differently. For instance, Nesta would have collaborated with more national partners, academic medical centers, laboratories, and accelerators. In India, Nesta is working with the Department of Biotechnology, which has an ecosystem of accelerators; the Longitude Prize would have benefited from participating in more arrangements like that, he said. It would also have been helpful to increase funding support through prototype development and validation, especially considering LMIC usability objectives, he added.

Berman suggested that the Longitude Prize would have benefited from being linked to a Carb-X initiative for maximum impact. Nesta has now established links with payers, but earlier involvement of potential payers and provider institutions could have been useful in steering developers toward priorities and deepening their understanding of clinical pathways. He added that the Longitude Prize would also have benefited from more advocacy to support increased biological testing in AMR.

Potential Antimicrobial Resistance Investment Fund

Berman concluded by challenging the current thinking about funding mechanisms. He said that the efforts to address the AMR crisis will fail unless a new or existing funding organization or mechanism can be effectively deployed. To that end, Nesta is encouraging the development of an AMR investment fund to catalyze innovation and develop a feasible market mechanism through a multistakeholder investment fund. Such a fund would call for new commitments from governments and institutions leading the AMR fight to facilitate innovation and overcome the failed market for antibiotics and diagnostics. Products could be funded based on WHO and member country priorities. Leadership by governments with support from development banks could be used to explore different mechanisms to finance the fund. Based on the antimicrobial investment fund's initial success, scale up could be achieved through G20 or other multilateral institutions, he added.

STRENGTHENING SYSTEMS TO OVERCOME BARRIERS TO INNOVATION

Jyoti Joshi explored how AMR efforts can be integrated into existing interventions and initiatives, and she discussed strategies to strengthen health systems and overcome market and regulatory barriers to innovation on AMR. She drew on her work with CDDEP, which is a small nonprofit think tank that works to bridge the gap between academia and implementation, including efforts to help address the complex challenge of AMR.

Global and National Action Plans for Antimicrobial Resistance

Joshi described the five pillars of WHO's Global Action Plan on Antimicrobial Resistance:

1. Developing awareness and understanding through communication, education, and training;
2. Building knowledge and evidence through AMR surveillance, laboratory science, and operational research;
3. Infection prevention and control in health care, animal health, food, and the community;
4. Optimizing use through regulation, antimicrobial stewardship, animal health, and agriculture; and

5. Investment, research, and development of new medicines and innovations (WHO, 2015).

She noted that the action plan is a policy document that does not yet have an integrated implementation footprint; many of the interventions under way are isolated, particularly in LMICs. CDDEP supports countries in tackling AMR by helping them to develop national action plans for AMR (NAP-AMR).

Joshi described a NAP-AMR as a "plan of plans" that is developed in collaboration with many country-level stakeholders, including government ministries, donors, nongovernmental organizations, and civil society. The planning process also involves consumers who take antibiotics, feed them to their animals, and ultimately ingest antibiotics that end up in water and sanitation systems. NAP-AMR plans are multisectoral and relate to numerous ministries in LMICs, including animal husbandry, health, population and family welfare, finance, human resources development, agriculture and farmers' welfare, and education and development.

Integrating Antimicrobial Resistance into Existing Interventions and Initiatives

Joshi explained that an AMR lens needs to be applied to existing interventions in order to address the AMR problem (WHO, 2018b, 2019g). AMR-specific interventions are those that specifically address the transmission of resistance through hospitals, humans, or animal–human interaction. These interventions strengthen components of health systems, agricultural systems, and environmental management of antibiotic use as well as introducing AMR and antimicrobial use surveillance and stewardship. AMR-sensitive interventions are primarily aimed at objectives other than AMR, but they indirectly help AMR containment. She noted that AMR-sensitive interventions that already exist in vertical programs can be intertwined. In this way, the AMR perspective can be used to identify and address gaps in funding for AMR-sensitive interventions. For example, AMR-sensitive interventions can increase capacity in health care, schools, households, and agriculture; they can contribute to scale up of infection prevention measures, such as improving UNICEF's[6] water, sanitation, and hygiene practices and extending vaccination of people and animals.

Joshi highlighted multiple existing entry points for AMR in existing initiatives and interventions. For instance, universal health coverage can provide a minimum services package for social insurance for all or select at-risk groups. Maternal and child health programs and the community-based

[6] Officially the United Nations Children's Fund, known as UNICEF.

Integrated Management of Childhood Illness provide opportunities to build awareness about AMR and stewardship in practice. Hospital-based quality-of-care programs and disease-specific programs (e.g., tuberculosis, malaria, HIV, and emerging zoonotic diseases) can also be used to build antibiotic stewardship and implement infection prevention and control activities to tackle AMR. Pooled procurement and generic drugs can help to ensure continuous access to quality-assured antimicrobials when needed, she added.

Barriers to Accessing Antibiotics

CDDEP published a report that identified three barriers to access to antibiotics based on scenarios in high-, middle-, and low-income settings, said Joshi (Frost et al., 2019). The first barrier is that weak drug discovery, difficulties in market entry, and poor stewardship lead to irrational selection and use of antibiotics. The second barrier is that antibiotics are not affordable for many in LMICs, and government funding for health is low. She pointed out that increasingly, AMR is a major cause of death in LMICs, yet more people in LMICs die from lack of access to antibiotics than from AMR, which creates further complications. The third barrier is that weak health systems, unreliable supply chains, and poor-quality control practices fail to deliver antibiotics to patients in need. The siloed nature of health systems and the poor management of supply chains make it difficult to ensure access to antibiotics in settings where they are needed, she added.

Joshi provided several findings from the report that exemplify these access barriers to antibiotics (Frost et al., 2019). Despite the availability of the vaccine, people die of *Streptococcus*-related meningitis or pneumonia around the world. The burden of gonococcal isolates with resistance to ciprofloxacin is greatest in countries that cannot afford to diagnose or treat people. Antibiotic consumption has risen in LMICs, even though the per capita consumption remains higher in the United States. For instance, the increase in per-capita antibiotic consumption in India is 300 times greater than in the United States. She noted that antibiotic prescription practices and the antibiotics prescribed vary worldwide; some countries have good-quality accreditation programs, but many LMICs do not. Additional challenges rise from the availability of antibiotics to consumers without prescription, she said. Although regulations require consumers to have prescriptions to obtain antibiotics, enforcement of these regulations has been a challenge. As a result, new chemical entities are not entering the market in places where they are most urgently needed.

Challenges in Harmonizing Antimicrobial Resistance Efforts

AMR control efforts are in different phases of evolution and management worldwide, Joshi noted. Harmonizing those efforts under the umbrella of One Health is a valuable goal, albeit one that will be difficult to achieve. Providing additional examples from the CDDEP report (Frost et al., 2019), Joshi noted that catastrophic health spending is a major challenge. Access to health care is among the primary limitations to containing AMR, yet most people in LMICs access health care through out-of-pocket expenditure. Unless good-quality, accredited, benchmarked care is provided through universal health coverage, access to health care will remain as a limitation for AMR efforts. Cost of care is another barrier, she said. Health care costs are immense in both LMICs and high-income countries. In Germany for example, the costs of second- and third-line antibiotics are much greater than the cost of first-line antibiotics, so uncomplicated infections are easier to treat.

Addressing Regulatory and Systemic Barriers to Foster Antimicrobial Resistance Innovation

Joshi discussed some of the regulatory barriers to innovation on AMR. The siloed approach to AMR interventions in human, animal, food, feed, and environmental sectors is a barrier to innovation, she remarked. As a result, there is a dearth of data connecting AMR with other types of interventions, such as the introduction of conjugate vaccines, that may have an effect on AMR. More data are also needed on the transmission of AMR through food chains, animals, and the environment, she added. More funding is needed for One Health sectors to undertake AMR interventions. Funding for drug discovery and stewardship is siloed and typically limited to funding research. Extending funds to implementation will require the appropriate plans, governance, and systems to be in place, however.

The regulatory capacity for monitoring animal and human antibiotic use, particularly the quality of antibiotic drugs, is another barrier to fostering innovation on addressing AMR. New drugs cannot be tested without sufficient funding, human resources, and laboratory capacity. She suggested that regulation and policy innovations that provide room for experimentation are needed to overcome these regulatory barriers.

Systems will need to be improved to reduce the barriers to research and development of novel antibiotics, said Joshi. Strategies for strengthening systems include innovative funding mechanisms for novel antibiotics and support for the registration of newly discovered molecules, as needed. In developing new antibiotics, registration should be factored into the planning and cost in addition to the discovery, research, and development phase. The antibiotic registration process should be aligned across national regulatory authorities to make it faster and simpler, she suggested. Mechanisms to monitor the quality of antibiotics are also needed. However, this will require strengthening drug regulatory capacity in LMICs, given that antibiotics can now be ordered online from countries around the world that may not have stringent regulatory and monitoring processes in place.

Health systems in LMICs will need to be strengthened to improve access and ensure appropriate use of antibiotics, said Joshi. This warrants a two-pronged approach to ensure that new molecules are accessible where they are needed and that the functions of existing molecules are retained and preserved. To achieve both of these aims, substantial investment will be needed to strengthen systems and foster collaboration across stakeholders (Gandra et al., 2017). Innovation of new molecules and preservation of current antibiotics will require collaboration across a broad range of stakeholders, including governments, national regulatory agencies, international agencies and donors, pharmaceutical industries and associations, clinical research organizations, distributors, retailers and pharmacists, logistics and supply chains, academia, and civil society.

Joshi added that funding will also be required to ensure that these systems are integrated, equitable, and sustainable in providing access to antibiotics, facilitating stewardship, and enforcing antibiotic prescription restrictions. She suggested that the AMR lens that is already being used in One Health approaches can also help to ensure that the appropriate balance is struck between access to effective treatment and protection from the overuse of antibiotics that promotes AMR.

DISCUSSION

Cristina Cassetti opened the discussion with her reflections on the panel presentations. She remarked that Johnson's presentation highlighted the importance of conducting surveillance in communities where people are in close contact with farm animals and wildlife. She commented that Kim's presentation revealed that there is much room for strengthening the development pipeline, and she noted Berman's acknowledgment of the need for earlier engagement with partners, payers, and downstream funders. Joshi's presentation identified the key barriers to innovation in AMR, highlighting the weak drug discovery pipeline, the difficulty of entering the markets, and poor stewardship of antibiotics, said Cassetti.

Peter Daszak asked Berman about the philosophy behind awarding the Longitude Prize to just a single winner and asked why the prize model is gaining traction over the more traditional grant-based method. Berman pointed out that grants tend to create an ecosystem in which it is possible to predict who will apply for them; competitions tend to bring in actors who otherwise would not have been involved. Berman suggested that this difference is a likely reason for the recent shift toward prize models. He acknowledged that the prize-based model leads to unhappy nonwinning teams; however, Nesta has distributed grants of as little as £25,000 to many of the competing teams. He also asserted that the true value of winning is not in the prize itself. Being the winner of a prize, such as the Longitude Prize, brings prestige and marketability that is a prize in and of itself. Furthermore, the judging panel and committee for the Longitude Prize consist of key actors in the space; thus, all teams benefit from having participated in terms of marketing and networking around highly specific global health objectives.

Greg Armstrong commented that the lack of investment in infection control is an additional barrier to fostering innovations on addressing AMR. Infection control is an orphaned problem in global health, and it is difficult to engage funders or governments in infection control, according to Armstrong; yet, infection control exacerbates AMR and puts patients and health care workers at serious risk for blood-borne and other pathogens. Joshi agreed and pointed out that there are limited data on the transmission dynamics of AMR in LMICs and a lack of investment in infrastructure elements, such as water and sanitation. The value of such investments for infection control is underappreciated because of the lack of data and research, but programs and governments do not have the ability to fund research on transmission dynamics of AMR. However, she noted that research is catching up in programs that promote quality of care and are the recipients of government investment.

John Gardinier, retired, National Center for Health Statistics, remarked on the inattention to negative results across scientific research. Kim reiterated that when Pew engages with potential data contributors, they do not request data from active programs; rather, they target programs that have been discontinued for any reason. This approach was informed by Pew's engagement in the community, which revealed that the same mistakes were being made repeatedly in antibiotics discovery research. The resources being directed into the antibiotic discovery field are diminishing, so there is a growing need to be more efficient with the approach to scientific discovery and to avoid repeating mistakes. In collecting data for SPARK from discontinued programs, Pew hopes to prevent labs from repeating mistakes that have already been made elsewhere.

Rick Bright, director, Biomedical Advanced Research and Development Authority, commented that like other major public health threats, AMR will require end-to-end innovation to work toward solutions. He maintained that there is no such thing as negative data. The innovation taking place within consortiums, incubators, accelerators, hubs, and other partnerships around the world have a responsibility to collect and share all data, because what seems like unsatisfactory endpoints for one particular goal might be the panacea for another. He noted the unique challenges associated with sharing data. Berman agreed that the issue of sharing data is of special concern in the field of antibiotic development. He mentioned the REVIVE project, developed by the Global Antibiotic Research and Development Partnership, which is intended to revive the area of antimicrobial discovery. He suggested that governments should take a proactive approach to creating paradigms for sharing data. For example, governments could create projects to fund milestones toward antibiotic development and then manage antibiotic development projects.

Kim added that Pew has engaged in discussions with government-funded programs in which the argument has been made that data from tax-funded research should be shared publicly. He suggested that a balance must be struck between the value proposition of intellectual property as a competitive advantage and the value of sharing data.

Marcos Espinal commented that he agreed with the panelists who called for the development for new products and compounds. However, he was concerned about how to protect new compounds as they are developed. AMR is a problem that has persisted since the advent of antibiotics, he noted, but the United Nations high-level meeting raised the stakes for AMR in a way that has driven interest and action. However, until governments take the initiative, the issues of AMR will continue to go unaddressed, and new antibiotics will be lost to resistance.

Espinal highlighted progress in the tripartite agreement among WHO, the Food and Agriculture Organization of the United Nations, and the World Organisation for Animal Health, as well as global and national action plans, but he noted that the action plans must be followed through to implementation to have an impact. He noted that in Latin America, countries have rules and laws that prohibit the sale of antibiotics without prescriptions, but these rules and laws are not enforced. Given the poor enforcement of policies regarding human health, he raised the question of how these concerns are being managed in animal health. He lauded the creation of multipartner trust funds but reiterated that the greatest challenge is protecting new products from AMR.

Berman suggested that the issues at the heart of Espinal's remarks are stewardship and demand, which are distinct from the issues and concerns around innovation. He agreed with Espinal's sentiment that the preferred approach to managing AMR is reducing demand and promoting stewardship and the rational use of antibiotics; however, it is also necessary to put focus on innovation, especially considering the amount of time required to develop new antibiotics. He agreed that there are development banks that are helping countries create stewardship programs and properly implement One Health, but innovation requires both push and pull funding that require separate financing streams.

Joshi added that the biggest challenge to the preservation of antibiotics is awareness, which is contingent on sociocultural norms that vary widely across settings. For example, in LMICs, it is not uncommon for a person to purchase antibiotics after 2 or 3 days of unresolved sickness without ever consulting a doctor, owing to costs of care and other cultural practices. Behavior change is required because the laws to prevent this activity are already in place. Best practices for implementing the necessary behavioral and enforcement changes have not been established, however. She suggested that those best practices need to be developed, tested, and scaled up as interventions in order to change the behaviors of consumers, practitioners, and dispensaries.

People need to understand that accessing antibiotics without a prescription is unethical and causes harm by accelerating resistance; this message needs to be appropriately packaged and delivered to the public. She also commented on the use of action plans. CDDEP worked with WHO to develop a guidance document on how to implement national plans, because many countries are not aware of how to do so. Implementing national AMR plans also helps in seeking funding, she added. For example, countries implementing vaccines need to have a plan for monitoring changes in transmission and resistance so their vaccination programs can be sustainable; these data can also be used to pitch for AMR funding.

Rafael Obregón asked whether PREDICT's social behavior dimension goes beyond the design and innovation development process and into implementation. Johnson explained that they made great efforts to bring social science and behavioral science expertise and approaches into their surveillance activities in each county where PREDICT worked. They investigated detailed quantitative questions related to human and animal activities in each setting, but they also collected qualitative social science data about cultural issues, such as the thoughts and beliefs of the community about interactions with animals, which were used to understand the communities' lens of zoonotic disease and inform interventions. PREDICT's findings have now been packaged around the human activities that potentially increase microbial threats. Obregón remarked that Joshi's recommendations for strengthening health systems did not include a recommendation regarding engaging communities and working around behavioral issues. He pointed out that the *Lancet Commission Report on Quality Health Systems* identified empowering consumers as a critical element, calling for an assessment of consumer levels of satisfaction and the assurance that consumers understand what quality means (Kruk et al., 2018). He noted that these issues also pertain to AMR. He asked how our understanding of how people engage with the ecosystem around antibiotics could be integrated into the overall approach to strengthening health systems in the context of AMR.

Joshi highlighted the importance of advocacy through communities, government regulations that leave room for experimentation, and policies that engage all stakeholders, including consumers, health care providers, and civil society. Health systems need to have resilience and preparedness built in, she explained. The challenges of AMR cannot be addressed through a one-time peak in awareness, like an "antibiotic awareness week." Instead, AMR needs to be incorporated into systematic, routine activities, such as infection prevention and control. She emphasized the importance of messaging around the consumption of antibiotics, which must be uniform across primary health care physicians and specialists. Health systems need to work toward co-creating clear, impactful messaging that is consistent and understood by children, parents, and health care providers alike. She asserted that appropriately addressing these issues is dependent on how activities are planned, funded, and implemented.

6

Breaking Down Barriers and Fostering Partnerships to Enable Innovation

The fourth session of the workshop, which focused on overcoming barriers and forging partnerships, was moderated by Alan Tennenberg, chief medical officer, Global Public Health, Johnson & Johnson. The session's objectives were to discuss novel strategies to enhance existing or stimulate new cross-sectoral collaborations and public–private partnerships, as well as to identify promising approaches to ensure the sustainability of innovative interventions. The session featured two panels, the first of which explored strategies for breaking down barriers and fostering new forms of partnership to enable innovation.

During the first panel, Colonel Matthew Hepburn, joint product lead, U.S. Army, discussed strategies for enabling biotechnologies through partnerships. Rahima Dosani, global health market access advisor, Center for Innovation and Impact, U.S. Agency for International Development (USAID), described her organization's approach to fostering new partnerships to enable innovation. Rajeev Venkayya, president, Global Vaccine Unit, Takeda Pharmaceuticals, remarked on opportunities for partnership models to address unmet needs in global health, particularly in low- and middle-income countries (LMICs). Tennenberg remarked that multisectoral collaboration is the only way to effectively counter the global health challenges being faced today. No sector can face these challenges alone, he said, but great things are possible when each sector brings its unique attributes to the table. However, lack of trust and poorly aligned objectives can threaten the success of those partnerships. He asked the panelists to consider how those barriers can be overcome to "beat back the pathogens at the gate."

ENABLING BIOTECHNOLOGIES THROUGH PARTNERSHIPS

Matthew Hepburn described a process for enabling biotechnologies through partnerships—"from information to injection." He leads a newly formed and integrated effort called the Joint Program Executive Office for Chemical, Biological, Radiological and Nuclear Defense (JPEO-CBRND).[1] The project focuses on the advanced development of biomedical products to solve infectious diseases and chemical, biological, radiological, and nuclear threats. Its aim is to develop medical solutions by enabling biotechnologies to facilitate rapid response during crises against future threats.

He explained that JPEO-CBRND is not responsible for the entire development of a product through its life cycle; rather, it works with partners with government, academia, and the private sector to accelerate products at steady state. He suggested that colleagues in the private sector and academia should consider JPEO-CBRND as an enabler of next-generation technology, rather than another entity seeking funds for product development. He added that JPEO-CBRND should receive the first call from the Secretary of Defense in a situation that warrants a medical solution to address an outbreak or threat for which there is no vaccine or therapeutic agent—or only preclinical products—that needs to be rolled out to thousands of people in a short period of time.

Strategies for Enabling Biotechnologies Through Partnerships

Hepburn pointed out that the mission of JPEO-CBRND is different from the mission of an organization such as the Biomedical Advanced Research and Development Authority (BARDA), which is tasked with protecting 350 million Americans. Instead, JPEO-CBRND's role is to be an early firebreak providing rapid deployment of vaccines or therapeutics while the larger national and international responses are gearing up. To do so, JPEO-CBRND concentrates on adopting next-generation technology and working through integrated partnerships from start to finish. Hepburn stated that the guiding premise of JPEO-CBRND is that during a crisis, the focus needs to be on the four components that have been reorganized within the U.S. Department of Defense (DoD) to accomplish this mission: (1) characterizing a threat, (2) selecting technology, (3) manufacturing a product, and (4) testing and distributing the product.

Characterizing the threat through global sample identification and sample characterization is carried out through partnerships as well as investments in biodetection assays and international sequencing programs, said

---

[1] Information about the Joint Program Executive Office for Chemical, Biological, Radiological and Nuclear Defense is available at https://www.jpeocbrnd.osd.mil (accessed February 8, 2020).

Hepburn. Through partnership with groups such as the U.S. Centers for Disease Control and Prevention and other groups in DoD, JPEO-CBRND aims to be at the forefront of making sequences available and understanding the emerging pathogen threat. He noted that academic centers tend to make sequencing information about pathogens available for antibody and vaccine discovery only after they publish the data. Hepburn maintained that this practice is not acceptable, because information about translating from sequence in real time is necessary for the medical product discovery process. JPEO-CBRND hopes to accomplish this in real time through integration and partnerships.

The next step is to select technology and accelerate product development. Hepburn explained that this step is intentionally referred to as "technology selection" rather than "discovery," because JPEO-CBRND focuses on partnerships to support existing products rather than reinventing the wheel. If no appropriate products are readily available, then JPEO-CBRND invests in automated antibody discovery. He highlighted a program run by the Defense Advanced Research Projects Agency (DARPA) called the Pandemic Prevention Platform, which invests in rapid antibody discovery against future pathogens. He remarked that this field is ripe and has reduced the timeline from years to weeks in terms of discovering a host of antibodies that could be useful against future pathogen threats. The challenge of selecting only a few from among the thousands of antibodies discovered to take into advanced development has the potential to be addressed by artificial intelligence and machine learning, he added.

The third component is manufacturing products and technology transfer through current good manufacturing practices, said Hepburn. DoD invested in an advanced development and manufacturing facility in Florida after the H1N1 pandemic in 2009, he continued. The facility is privately owned, but it is linked with a network at BARDA to provide surge capacity in a crisis. Hepburn said that as soon as JPEO-CBRND has a product available—even while the discovery process is still ongoing—the product immediately goes to the front of the line for manufacturing and production at the facility.

The fourth component is to test products for safety and efficacy prior to distribution, said Hepburn. The capacity to conduct clinical trials is being built out further with DoD's aim to improve the ability to have mobile and global outbreak clinical trial capabilities. As an example, Hepburn commended the Congolese volunteers and colleagues from the National Institutes of Health and the World Health Organization, who demonstrated that a randomized controlled trial can be conducted in Ebola treatment units in a conflict zone during a crisis, dispelling the notion that clinical trials are not feasible during an outbreak. He highlighted the need to adopt next-generation technologies, including electronic data capture and continuous physiologic monitoring. He added that DoD needs these next-generation technologies to deliver prolonged field care for its worldwide deployed force.

FOSTERING NEW PARTNERSHIPS TO ENABLE INNOVATION

Building on Hepburn's discussion of the importance of partnerships, Rahima Dosani described USAID's overall approach to private-sector partnerships, provided examples of successful partnerships, and suggested a set of best practices for creating and sustaining effective cross-sectoral partnerships.

USAID's Approach to Private-Sector Engagement

Private-sector engagement is critical to USAID's global health work to combat microbial threats, said Dosani (USAID, 2019a,b). Cross-sectoral partnerships are needed because the public sector cannot address those threats on its own. Traditional grant funding will not be sufficient to meet the health-related United Nations Sustainable Development Goals (SDGs) given the $134 billion investment gap for health-related SDGs in LMICs, which is expected to triple to $371 billion in the next 10 years (Stenberg et al., 2017). She described the private sector as a significant source of incredible networks, systems, and technical expertise, as well as an increasingly significant source of providing services in LMICs. For example, in many countries, the majority of people who seek care for fevers do so in the private sector (Ansah et al., 2016). Collaborations with the private sector offer contributions in technical expertise, networks, strategic systems, and flexibility, she added.

USAID's perspective is that the future of development will primarily be enterprise driven and reliant on private-sector collaboration, said Dosani. Business as usual will not end the need for assistance; private-sector engagement is needed to foster collaboration with the private sector, make catalytic use of USAID resources, seek market-based solutions for greater sustainability, and mobilize private capital for scale. She shared several private-sector engagement principles developed by USAID:

- To engage early and often with private-sector actors and other partners to design and implement strategies and projects of shared value;
- To incentivize and value private-sector engagement throughout planning and programming to adapt continuously to new evidence, opportunities, or circumstances;
- To expand the use of USAID approaches and tools that unlock the potential of the private sector; and

- To build and act on the evidence of what works and what does not work.

Over USAID's long history of building partnerships, it has found that private-sector partnerships can catalyze health goals to scale to be efficient, cost-effective, and sustainable, said Dosani. Increasing scale enables programs to reach more of the target population by drawing on private-sector resources and expertise or by accessing private-sector channels (USAID, 2019b). Greater efficiency involves operating more efficiently or cost-effectively by adapting private-sector expertise, skills, or tools. Private-sector partnerships also improve cost-effectiveness by achieving procurement savings from more competitive markets that facilitate access to health products and open or expand markets for commercial actors. Program sustainability can be enhanced by using handover strategies, revenue-generating business models, and commercially viable, local private-sector partners. To illustrate these advantages, Dosani shared three examples of USAID's successful private-sector partnerships, which have evolved through various stages of success and lack thereof (see Box 6-1).

BOX 6-1
Examples of the U.S. Agency for International Development's (USAID's) Successful Private-Sector Partnerships

The Aspen Management Partnership for Health (AMP Health) uses a variety of private-sector partnerships to increase the leadership capacity of government ministries of health. They work with ministries of health to build effective leadership and management practices by leveraging private-sector skills and expertise. As an example of the high efficiency and leverage of USAID investments, AMP Health attracted $1.2 million in private-sector funds and an additional $1.3 million in philanthropic funds to extend impact of $0.8 million in USAID investment in this area.

The UBS Optimus Foundation and Merck for Mothers brought in private-sector capital to create a development impact bond to address the quality of private-sector facilities in India and improve maternal and child health outcomes. USAID worked with the UBS Optimus Foundation on the Utkrisht Development Impact Bond to accredit private providers to offer quality maternal and neonatal health services, while UBS provided working capital for accreditation. Only after the quality threshold is reached do USAID and Merck pay for quality outcomes.

Project Last Mile and Coca-Cola used the latter's expertise to improve supply chains and improve access to lifesaving medicines and supplies at the "last mile" of African nations through supply chain and strategic marketing support. This project has enrolled 2 million HIV-positive patients in a South African program for convenient drug pickups.

Practices to Create and Sustain Effective Cross-Sectoral Partnerships

Using the example of work by the Aspen Management Partnership for Health (AMP Health) to increase the leadership capacity of government ministries of health, Dosani highlighted a set of best practices for creating and sustaining effective cross-sectoral, private-sector partnerships. The first is that private-sector engagement can take many forms and should be iterative; the second is that interests should be aligned and each partner's unique assets should be leveraged; and the third is that progress should be measured early to track impact, and lessons from mistakes should be used to inform and evolve the partnership over time.

Spectrum of Private-Sector Engagement Options

Dosani explained that a spectrum of private-sector engagement options exists, with different types of engagement involving different amounts of risk and investment. In a government-led engagement, government is the driver in leveraging private-sector resources and expertise; this type of engagement may or may not be aligned with commercial interests or core business operations. In co-creation, the government is a co-creator engaged with the private sector jointly identifying challenges and designing programming to address shared interests; this includes the co-creation of market-based approaches. In private-sector-led engagement, the government is the facilitator in providing assistance in addressing private-sector constraints and risks; these engagements may be built on for-profit and market-based approaches to challenges.

She noted that private-sector engagements are iterative and do not necessarily lead to formal, full-on partnerships. For example, a private-sector entity can be engaged to co-create a target product profile, test products during research and development, or consider how to bring a product or service to scale. Partnerships start with light touch engagement during an early stage of exploration and can move into a curated stage where engagement is refined, with each partner having set work streams with defined goals. If a strong model of partnership is identified, the proof-of-concept stage includes a pilot project to test the value and impact of collaboration. In the case that a best model of partnership has been identified and piloted—with clear value and impact for all collaborators—then the model can be further tested through scale in other environments or countries. Areas for consideration at each stage of partnership include the potential impact and time until execution, the assessment of risk, the level of government effort, and the level of commitment from the private sector. She added that the same considerations apply at each stage of engagement, but the bar for risk and certain impact gets higher as progress is made.

Aligning Interests and Finding Shared Value

Dosani's second best practice for private-sector engagement was to align interests and find shared value. The engagement archetype ought to be based on shared interests. In the first stage of exploration, she remarked, the goals for the public sector are achieving effective coverage, quality, cost-efficiency, and sustainability; for the private sector, the goals are growth, risk diversification, public relations with the government and community, and having a healthy workforce. She highlighted four different project archetypes: corporate philanthropy, corporate social responsibility, shared interest, and investment. In the execution phase, private-sector engagement activities should be designed to achieve shared interests and make a health impact. In the supporting-to-scale phase, long-term commitment from both the government and the partner should be confirmed. At each stage, Dosani advised questioning whether the appropriate approach is being used.

Dosani linked these practices to the partnership with AMP Health, which has a diverse set of partners that has catalyzed exponential rather than linear results. Through a range of public, private, and nonprofit partnerships, it has been successful in teaching many new skills and approaches in the past 4 years. She pointed out that AMP Health places management partners within a certain team for at least 2 years to help build the capacity of its teams. It has successfully aligned the interests of the three pharmaceutical companies that have supported them; this enables teams to make better and more strategic choices about resource allocation, which aligns in the best interests of the pharmaceutical companies as well. This holistic, team-based approach includes management partners, but also extends to in-country workshops and live learning, distance learning, one-on-one executive coaching, focus work streams, and leadership labs.

AMP Health also rigorously evaluates its impact, she said. This is conducted through the following:

- Regular measurement of an individual's development of leadership and management capabilities;
- Regular measurement of team effectiveness;
- Keeping scorecards of leadership and management best practices, tools, and processes used by high-functioning teams;
- Tracking and describing concurrent health system evolution; and
- Undertaking qualitative measurement of the leadership and management journey.

Adapting and Evolving Partnership Models

Dosani highlighted the importance of learning from failure and continuously adapting and evolving partnership models. For instance, AMP Health has evolved and made organizational changes in response to past mistakes. Specifically, after an initial partnership in Kenya, AMP Health decided not to continue work with the community health team at the Ministry of Health because of devolution and political challenges. As the political landscape changed, AMP Health realized that it was not an adapting and enabling context for its work. AMP Health is completely demand driven and only works in countries and departments within ministries of health where there is a direct government request for partnership. Instead of providing traditional technical assistance, it focuses on building the capacity of entire teams. It supports ministries of health longitudinally, guided by the idea that achieving long-lasting behavior change and building capacity takes time and commitment beyond short funding cycles, she added.

PRIVATE-SECTOR PARTNERSHIPS TO ADDRESS GLOBAL HEALTH NEEDS

Rajeev Venkayya drew on his range of experiences with the Coalition for Epidemic Preparedness Innovations (CEPI) as a grant recipient from major international funding bodies, and as a contract recipient from BARDA to reflect on some of the opportunities and challenges in forging private-sector partnerships to address unmet global health needs. Venkayya remarked that the partnership model needed to conduct mission-driven research to address major unmet needs in global health in LMICs is complex. The industry has a long track record of developing products for developed markets, but innovation is needed to encourage the development of products for those markets that are not as attractive for private-sector entities.

He clarified that there is industry interest in supporting the needs of developing markets, but companies are accountable to stockholders and investors and need to demonstrate that the capital invested in product development will have a return that is competitive with other opportunities. These companies have expertise in developing these types of products that need to be developed for LMICs in order to create a greater probability of success, he added.

Opportunities for Partnership to Strengthen the Vaccine Clinical Development Cycle

Venkayya considered strategies for optimizing and strengthening the partnership model around the clinical development cycle for vaccines, from candidate vaccines to licensed vaccines that can be used in the field. For many diseases faced in LMICs—such as Lassa fever, Middle East respiratory syndrome (MERS), Nipah virus, and chikungunya—there is no shortage of vaccine candidates. In CEPI's efforts to find partners, it has found many entities interested in developing these vaccines, but fewer who have experience in taking vaccines all the way through to development and licensure. He said that compared to the early stages of vaccine development, CEPI and other large industry partners can play a more substantial role during the later stages of vaccine development.

During the later stages, vaccine development is a risky, capital-intensive, and lengthy process because the high bar for safety and efficacy requires large clinical trials that can pick up low or infrequently occurring adverse effects that need to be identified before large-scale deployment of a vaccine. For example, the dengue vaccine program is currently being evaluated in a phase 3 trial that has enrolled 20,000 children across 8 countries. The hope is that this trial may have enough dengue patients to demonstrate a statistically significant effect of the vaccine in groups of individuals that require it.

Further challenges relate to demonstrating efficacy, particularly when the population that will be exposed to the infectious agent is unknown and huge populations need to be immunized in order to ensure that certain numbers are exposed to the threat and placebo in the vaccine group. In addition to those barriers, the chemistry, manufacturing, and controls requirements around process development and validation drive the substantial expense and time associated with vaccine development, he said.

Venkayya suggested that a strategy to address barriers related to expense and timelines of vaccine development is to determine correlates of protection—meaning, identifying factors that will accurately predict the protection and the deployment of the vaccine into large populations. This would be helpful for vaccines against dengue, chikungunya, and other emerging infectious diseases. Another opportunity is to develop pathways that are predictable enough to allow the licensure of vaccines without large-scale efficacy trials. Sometimes called "accelerated review pathways," these rely primarily on preclinical and clinical data that demonstrate certain levels of antibodies that correlate with protection in animal models, which will then lead to licensure with substantial postmarketing commitments. He added that this type of pathway would also unlock efficiencies and reduce costs in vaccine development. Venkayya maintained that the burden should not be placed on regulators alone. Companies have a role to play because they understand what is required to develop their products, and they should provide regulators with ideas about how to reconsider the regulatory pathway to licensure.

Challenges in Engaging the Private Sector to Address Global Health Needs

Venkayya described how CEPI is tackling the issue of unmet needs in global health by engaging the private sector. The challenge for large companies considering involvement in these types of programs goes beyond technical risk to substantial market risks. These include whether there will be the epidemiology to support uptake of the vaccine if it is successfully developed and licensed as well as vaccine hesitancy concerns. Other risks relate to the margin differences among low-, middle-, and high-income countries, which are associated with tiered pricing, which fundamentally change the risk and investment dynamic in companies. He highlighted push funding as an easy solution demonstrated by CEPI, the Bill & Melinda Gates Foundation, and product development partnerships. Push funding decreases the risk for companies and incentivizes them to accept the opportunity cost of deploying their resources from more predictable programs to one that has a different risk and investment profile, he noted. For instance, BARDA is providing Takeda Pharmaceuticals with cost reimbursement that allows the company to address public health challenges, such as Zika.

Ideological Concerns in Private-Sector Partnerships

Venkayya noted that there are ideological issues in the ecosystem around public–private partnerships to achieve product development goals: concern and trepidation that public funds are going to companies that are perceived to have significant resources to develop products for the public good, but that those products will not be accessible after they are developed. He surmised that this fear may be driven by situations in which the pricing of products for HIV has made them inaccessible. However, he said that the companies who seek out engagement with entities like CEPI are doing so because they genuinely want to address public health problems.

Venkayya sees social media and other media as mechanisms of accountability to apply pressure to companies that have taken public funds to develop a product for the public good but do not act appropriately. He described this as an "insurance policy" to ensure that groups like CEPI are partnering with companies that will do what is necessary from an access standpoint. He added that the most important element of a strong partnership between industry and funding entities is trust, which spans the dimensions of competency, honesty, and benevolence (Grayson, 2016). For example, BARDA has confidence that Takeda knows what it is doing, that it can deliver on a product, that it will be transparent, and that it is in the partnership in order to do the "right thing." Venkayya suggested that these dimensions need to be rigorously applied to all partnerships and private-sector engagements.

DISCUSSION

Tennenberg remarked that CEPI is a strong example of partnership between multiple stakeholders to tackle public health needs and asked about how the organization came into existence. Venkayya said that it involved the efforts of hundreds of people and organizations such as the National Academies of Sciences, Engineering, and Medicine. The 2014 Ebola epidemic was a driver of CEPI, because there were vaccines in the pipeline but no framework with which to evaluate the vaccines quickly in the field. CEPI took on the challenge of looking at the highest epidemic threats in the world and investing in a pipeline to bring vaccine candidates up to phase 2A or 2B, so that phase 3–ready compounds could be deployed into the field with appropriate clinical trials when an epidemic emerges. He noted that this was the original model, but it would be very complex to follow this template in reality, so he expects modifications going forward.

Venkayya added that CEPI has been successful in implementing a broad range of partnerships that have contributed to a broad range of vaccine candidates in the pipeline. Brian Bird said he previously worked on developing a vaccine for Rift Valley fever that was recently selected by CEPI for further development in their human pipeline. He remarked that CEPI brought a wealth of expertise to the technical side of the process that was also beneficial from a funding agency's perspective. He suggested applying this type of collaborative approach to antimicrobial resistance and other seemingly intractable problems.

Tennenberg pointed out the "elephant in the room" of large health care companies needing to answer to shareholders, remaining accountable to the business plan, and maintaining their top and bottom lines. He asked for strategies to motivate companies to be involved in projects with a return on investment that will be lower than other opportunities. Hepburn said that when he was at DARPA, the model was to invest in the best people in the world to solve the problem, whether they were domestic, international, a small biotechnical company, a university, or part of cost-share partnerships with large pharmaceutical companies. He saw the advantages and disadvantages of working with each type of group, but a common issue was that the U.S. government does not negotiate very well for grants or cost-share partnerships. He suggested that negotiation should aim to achieve practical mutual benefit rather than the government simply providing money. He noted that the U.S. government has improved over the past decade in adopting new and different ways to contract these types of investments with small biotechnical and large pharmaceutical companies.

In cases where the opportunity cost for a company would be excessive, he suggested that the government should consider what else it can offer from its toolbox, such as adopting next-generation technology for clinical trials or cost sharing on testing a mutually beneficial vaccine using DoD's global network of clinical trials. Hepburn added that DoD and the U.S. Food and Drug Administration (FDA) have a strong relationship, which has been codified in public law, that works for the unique needs related to military medicine and infectious diseases. He suggested the potential for cost-share partnerships on vaccines with DoD and FDA, because private-sector input into regulatory policy is critical.

Dosani remarked that the return on investment is not necessarily as low as it is assumed to be—for instance, the development impact bond with the UBS Optimus Foundation and Merck has up to an 8 percent return—and there is a broad spectrum of ways these types of investments can provide good returns. Furthermore, negotiations to determine what both parties want out of the partnership may reveal that employees are interested in investing in social causes rather than financial interests. She added that negotiations with private-sector companies should seek to understand their interests and show that there is shared value in improving the company's operations as well.

Venkayya underscored the importance of being flexible and sophisticated in understanding what a partner specifically values. With respect to ideological issues around access, he noted that the Bill & Melinda Gates Foundation's global access policy was pioneering in its focus on getting products for populations in LMICs, which has now expanded to ensure that poor populations in middle- and upper-income countries are also benefiting from the investment. He added that allowing private entities to capture value in other markets with a platform that a funder has helped to develop or reduce risk is an example of how flexibility can engage the private sector while allowing the funder to achieve its aims as well.

Keiji Fukuda, director and clinical professor, The University of Hong Kong School of Public Health, commented on the difficulty in establishing public–private partnerships and asked how interests should be aligned among multiple partners in the context of a lack of trust and differing motives. He noted that although there are ad hoc partnerships and larger-scale entities such as CEPI, a larger ecosystem of partnership does not yet exist, perhaps owing to the focus on the private-sector side rather than the benefits of leadership, governance, and legitimacy that the public-sector side has to offer. Venkayya responded that CEPI still needs to make progress in engaging with large private-sector companies in vaccine development programs, but it is providing the elements of public-sector leadership, governance, and legitimacy. He suggested that this could be codified into a more predicable framework or structure through a coalition of like-minded partners, for example, as long as the framework also allows room to bring in external innovation.

Hepburn added that the government can provide leadership and legitimacy in addition to funding. He suggested that leadership at the highest level of government needs to advocate for more resources to support the public sector and develop a stronger ecosystem of partnerships. Dosani added that the public sector needs to be more intentional in carving out the time to create this type of ecosystem.

George Haringhuizen asked about enabling preparedness and fast response of mobile and global trials and materials data analysis and whether they are creating agreements in advance about access and benefit sharing with other countries. Hepburn replied that progress is being made, and the U.S. government generally does a good job of engaging with international organizations and partner countries in global health responses, but there is more work to be done.

Hepburn said that from a DoD standpoint, partnership with the host country is paramount; data are frequently shared, and they ensure that local partners receive first authorship on academic collaborations. DoD works to ensure that host countries benefit from the clinical trials and products being developed, but the complexity of these negotiations makes them challenging. He added that DoD benefits on a daily basis from opportunities for mutually beneficial military-to-military collaborations with North Atlantic Treaty Organization (NATO) allies and host countries to support health care delivery and public health emergency responses.

Peter Daszak commended the work by CEPI and other emerging initiatives around the pipeline for pathogens, but he noted that they depend on fragile partnerships and funding structures. He asked how USAID addresses sustainability within its public–private partnership initiatives, particularly in the context of political shifts. Dosani responded that ensuring sustainability is an ongoing challenge, given the fragility of partnerships. She added that many partnerships are not sustainable because it is challenging to track and quantify their impact. Starting to track and measure impact early in the process can help to improve sustainability by demonstrating the benefits of the work being done by the partnership.

Venkayya pointed out that CEPI is still an experiment that needs to demonstrate its success; this will take years owing to the timeline for vaccine development, so milestones needed to be added along the way to give donors confidence that it is on track. He was optimistic about CEPI's success, despite the challenges inherent in product development. For instance, many product development programs are guaranteed to fail, given the low likelihood of a given product making it to the market, and donors need to be willing to tolerate that outcome. He added that leadership and continuous assessment are important in ensuring that donors maintain confidence in the initiative.

Turkan Gardenier, applied statistician, asked about the application of geographical information science technology. Hepburn responded that the approach to clinical trials needs to be adapted to take into account the huge amount of information that is now available by using more sophisticated statistical design and analysis. He suggested that trials could possibly be carried out more quickly and with far fewer participants if cutting-edge data science and technology were applied—for example, using accurate point-of-care diagnostics to determine which patients have an infection in a therapeutic trial. Transforming the product development process could also reduce costs enormously, he added.

Jay Siegel, retired, asked whether the four-stage process presented by Hepburn was about monoclonal antibody development for therapeutics, passive immunization, or diagnostics. He also asked about the timeline from receiving a new pathogen to having a promising therapeutic and the extent to which partners are involved in the process. Hepburn responded that he used antibody development as the example because it is a promising technology. Furthermore, the pharmaceutical industry has reduced its risk, and there is a set process on how to make, test, manufacture, and license a monoclonal antibody. However, the same vision of rapid product development could be applied to vaccines.

He said that discovery is not the problem at this point—the back end of manufacturing and clinical trials is the primary challenge. He suggested that the best strategy for success during a crisis is minimal change, that is, to do everything by the same process that regulatory agencies are comfortable with at a steady rate. This strategy is starting to be used for antibody production as well as in various vaccine platforms, he noted, and expressed hope that it would streamline manufacturing and regulatory processes.

Jyoti Joshi pointed out that the private sector is not one player, but multiple players that are at different levels with distinct knowledge and expertise. She asked about how to balance concerns about safety in the context of accelerated introductions and review pathways, given that reports of product performance may be delayed in settings with health systems that are already weaker or easily compromised by an outbreak. More broadly, she asked how health systems' resilience and trust building figure into these conversations.

Venkayya said that when the Bill & Melinda Gates Foundation was introducing the rotavirus vaccine into LMICs, they considered the number of lives lost per day that the introduction of the vaccine was delayed. He suggested applying the same concept to product development timelines and urgency for epidemic diseases. The benefits of shortening timelines through alternative review and licensure pathways need to be weighed against safety concerns, however. This requires a benefit–risk calculation that takes into account management of risk on the safety and efficacy side as well as careful pharmacovigilance and safety monitoring once the product is released.

Accelerated access to the market is contingent on a robust set of postmarketing commitments to evaluate for safety, he added. It is possible to take a risk-based approach to the licensure pathway to accelerate product delivery, while also pacing the rollout to identify safety issues as the product is scaled. Hepburn suggested leveraging the power of next-generation technology, such as cell phones, to capture postmarketing safety data. He also called for using technology to democratize clinical trial enrollment and the capture of health care information, while ensuring that patients' private data are protected.

Carolyn Carroll, statistician, asked how to incorporate the risk profile into funding for new vaccines (e.g., the risks associated with Zika and Ebola). Venkayya responded that there are flavors of risk with any vaccine. Zika vaccine development, for example, had significant epidemiological and market risks. For a venture-backed or public company, the value proposition on a risk-adjusted basis of investing in a Zika vaccine is not attractive relative to other places that capital could be allocated. Takeda was willing to make the investment and take the risk because BARDA reduced the risk of the effort by shouldering much of the investment. Takeda still bears opportunity costs and other costs, but it is contributing to the vaccine development for the benefit of public health.

Rick Bright commented on the importance of trust, communication, and transparency in public–private partnerships, both from the bottom up and the top down. He also highlighted the discrepancy in interpreting the return on investment by different partners as the partnership evolves over time. For example, private entities may look at public funding as a gift or grant, while government entities such as BARDA are accountable for getting the full agreed-upon return on investment on behalf of the U.S. taxpayers, which, it is hoped, will benefit global public health as well. He added that BARDA has changed its approach to partnering with private industry to replace rigid, outdated contractual terms and to move toward flexible agreements that allow the government to behave more as a business partner in negotiations and discussions about return on investment.

Bright also highlighted innovation in regulatory sciences led by agencies such as FDA and the European Medicines Agency in terms of future drug production, vaccine development, and diagnostics. Venkayya noted an asymmetry in relationships between a funder and a contract or grant awardee. Awardees may not have the capability to aggregate risks in a sophisticated way and may face pressure to overpromise. He suggested that both sides of a partnership need to be more careful and candid about risks, timelines, and budgets.

Kent Kester remarked on the potential to look across technologies and platforms in the interagency world to focus on public health imperatives, codify best practices, and thus simplify and streamline the development of public–private partnerships. Hepburn said that DoD, USAID, and the U.S. Department of Health and Human Services are working together better than ever before, sharing research capacity and expertise. However, relationships and trust still need to be strengthened. He suggested focusing on building more formalized structures to codify best practices and ensure that this coordination outlasts individual relationships.

Daniel Berman suggested using negotiation and advanced market commitments or service contracts to generate public support for increased investment in partnerships for product development. Venkayya replied that prices should not be negotiated at the preclinical or phase 1 stage of development, because there are so many uncertainties that will have an effect on the price. However, it is possible to negotiate on the principles of how to operate, which CEPI is doing. He added that having donors and investors on the board adds layers of protection that help to ensure the appropriate use of taxpayer dollars and adherence to access provisions. CEPI has also put other mechanisms in place as a fallback to protect donor and taxpayer resources, as well as the populations that CEPI intends to help.

James Lawler, director, Clinical and Biodefence Research, National Strategic Research Institute, University of Nebraska, remarked that the products and technologies developed through these partnerships are not used in a vacuum; therefore, it is important to consider the effect they are actually having in practice. For example, new products being employed to address the Ebola outbreak in the Democratic Republic of the Congo are not having a substantial effect on the case fatality ratio. He suggested a focus on leveraging partnerships and investment to integrate high-quality supportive clinical care in resource-limited settings.

Hepburn acknowledged the tension between a focus on physical product development and adopting a holistic approach to outbreak response. He suggested that clinical trials for product development could be layered on top of an observational study to promote a more comprehensive understanding of health and disease during outbreaks. Eva Harris called for more discussion around governments, industry, and populations in the Global South and their roles as partners.

Dosani responded that USAID is focused on building countries' self-reliance, so partnerships are done in-country and led, to some extent, by country governments and are supported, rather than controlled at the agency level. The examples she discussed are supported by local governments, local nonprofits, and the local private sector. Andrew Clements, deputy director, Pandemic Influenza and Other Emerging Threats Unit, USAID, commented that in addition to biomedical inventions, there are other valuable preventive measures—such as infection prevention and control, water and sanitation, and livestock value chain biosecurity—that could benefit from partnerships with the private sector.

7

Nurturing Innovations Through Novel Ecosystems to Accelerate Research and Development

The second panel of the workshop's fourth session explored strategies for incubating research and development through novel ecosystems; it was moderated by Rick Bright, director, Biomedical Advanced Research and Development Authority (BARDA). Panelists discussed the key environmental features of novel ecosystems that enable innovations to tackle microbial threats. Sabrina Welsh, director of programs and operations, Human Vaccines Project, discussed the model of collaboration used by the Human Vaccines Project to broaden the understanding of the immune system in order to accelerate innovation.

Maurizio Vecchione, executive vice president of Global Good and Research, Intellectual Ventures, explored the concept of reverse innovation as a radical approach to forging public–private partnerships and developing ecosystems of innovation. Sally Allain, head, JLABS, described Johnson & Johnson Innovation's model of nurturing innovation to accelerate research and development. Ranga Sampath, chief scientific officer, Foundation for Innovative New Diagnostics (FIND), focused on the need to spur innovation in diagnostic tools.

BIOMEDICAL ADVANCED RESEARCH AND DEVELOPMENT AUTHORITY

Rick Bright commenced the panel by remarking that in many cases, "we are still using yesterday's technology to fight yesterday's challenges, but we are also using yesterday's technology to try to fight today's challenges." He noted that a pandemic scenario underscores the potential impact of failing to implement innovations that have been developed. Needles and syringes have been used to deliver vaccines since the first mass vaccination campaign against smallpox in the 1800s. Although investment has supported innovation in vaccination administration that could reduce cost, improve efficiency, and allow for a more rapid and accessible response, those innovations have not been implemented. Consequently, in a scenario of pandemic influenza, it is unlikely that the United States would be able to acquire and deploy hundreds of millions of vaccine doses quickly enough to stay in front of the pandemic, said Bright. Furthermore, he noted that it would probably take about 3 years for the United States to manufacture enough needles and syringes to administer the vaccine nationwide in a pandemic scenario.

Bright also reflected on his experience working with BARDA, which was established in 2006 to adopt a novel approach to fulfilling the promise of bridging government and industry within an intentionally designed organization. BARDA's mission is to form public–private partnerships to develop and accelerate the development of medical countermeasures to protect people from the greatest threats faced today. BARDA's collaboration with the National Institute of Allergy and Infectious Diseases, the U.S. Food and Drug Administration (FDA), the U.S. Centers for Disease Control and Prevention, and industry partners has contributed to an increase in the number of FDA-approved products over the past several years, he said. However, approved products such as vaccines that just sit in a vial or warehouse are completely ineffective.

Large amounts of investment are channeled into developing drugs or vaccines without commensurate investment in methods to accelerate and improve drug development or in systems to support the administration of products—particularly in the last mile of care. He observed that the road in that last mile and the vehicles used to get there have also changed over the years, and they will continue to evolve. New consortiums and partnerships will be necessary to create a future-oriented ecosystem and culture that can address the last mile in the future, he said. Without a forward-looking culture and ecosystem, there may be an erosion of the progress that has been made in the past.

To help BARDA change the way it does business beyond simply creating public–private partnerships, Bright travels extensively to experience innovation and entrepreneurship within the industry firsthand. This motivated him to establish a new division of BARDA called the Division of Research, Innovation, and Ventures,[1] along with a venture capital fund to stimulate investment of government funding in these areas.

---

[1] For more information on BARDA's Division of Research, Innovation, and Ventures (DRIVe), see https://drive.hhs.gov (accessed March 3, 2020).

DECODING THE HUMAN IMMUNE SYSTEM TO TRANSFORM HUMAN HEALTH

Sabrina Welsh's presentation explored how decoding the human immune system has the potential to transform the future of human health. She discussed the model of collaboration used by the Human Vaccines Project, a nonprofit public–private partnership with a large network of global collaborators. The Human Vaccines Project's mission is to broaden the understanding of the immune system and to accelerate the development of therapeutics, diagnostics, and vaccines for major global diseases.

A Paradigm Shift in Research and Development

The established research and development system is proving poorly suited to today's problems, said Welsh. The diseases being battled are more complex and evasive than in the past, especially with the rise of resistant microbes, and the traditional research and development paradigm does not move quickly enough to address these needs. Welsh highlighted a number of late-stage vaccine and immunotherapy failures for infectious diseases (e.g., HIV, tuberculosis, malaria, dengue) and noted that many noncommunicable diseases, such as cancers and autoimmune diseases, are lacking broadly effective treatment options.

Limitations in effectiveness are another challenge, she said. Many currently licensed vaccines are not effective in the most vulnerable populations, such as infants and older adults. Vaccines often require multiple immunizations and have limited durability. Immunotherapy works only for a small subset of cancer patients, leaving a large gap in treatment options. Research and development is a hugely expensive and lengthy process, yet the probability of success is low, she added. Animal models are not always good proxies for predicting how a candidate will respond in humans. Additionally, the resources required for vaccine research and development are in the range of $1 billion over decades.

Welsh considered why some people respond better than others to vaccines and therapeutics. Vaccine response is variable across vaccines and populations. Longitudinal data on measles, rubella, diphtheria, tetanus, and vaccinia vaccines demonstrate that the magnitude of antibody responses in individuals can vary by 10–200-fold. Some people respond immediately and achieve protection with a single dose; others may achieve partial protection with many doses or never achieve protection at all. Vaccination outcomes are also variable, she stated. For example, some people exposed to Ebola become infected, develop Ebola disease right away, and become symptomatic. Others exposed to Ebola may be asymptomatic or experience less severe disease symptoms. This variability has also been observed in HIV outcomes, in which some people's disease progression is rapid and others—called elite controllers—are able to control their viral load and stay asymptomatic for long periods of time.

HIV is a good example of the challenges faced in vaccine development that illustrates why a new approach is necessary, she noted. The virus and its weaknesses are well understood, and how a neutralizing antibody could block HIV from replicating or infecting has already been established. Even with this knowledge, an effective vaccine that elicits broadly neutralizing antibodies has not yet been developed.

New Approach to Understanding the Human Immune System

Lack of understanding of the human immune system is impeding development of new and improved vaccines, diagnostics, and therapies for major diseases, said Welsh. The key to a new approach, Welsh remarked, lies in unlocking the inner workings of the immune system. A convergence of technological advancements has created an unprecedented opportunity to harness the power of the immune system in the fight against disease. The Human Vaccines Project is taking an interdisciplinary approach by coupling advanced tools, systems biology, computational biology, bioinformatics, artificial intelligence (AI), and machine learning to gain a more comprehensive understanding of how the human immune system functions (Human Vaccines Project, 2020).

In the past, science has largely been organized into silos focused on individual diseases or specific components of disease. The Human Vaccines Project is using a different model that involves working across sectors and diseases and sharing data with the whole field. Its approach works within a network of scientific leaders from top universities, nonprofits, government, and industry to tackle multiple diseases and to examine immunology as a system.

By examining immunology as a system, the Human Vaccines Project intends to innovate and accelerate the development of products across the board, said Welsh. No single institution has the capacity to conduct this work independently, so the Human Vaccines Project has adopted a collaborative model to drive transformational leaps instead of incremental steps. The Human Vaccines Project's model includes transparent data sharing through a bioinformatics hub, guided by a stepwise data-sharing policy that includes specific timings for when data are to be released, uploaded, and available for access. The policy varies depending on the type of data being shared, she added.

The Human Vaccines Project has also developed a set of data standards and templates to enable data to be integrated and analyzed with the tools it has developed and made available, Welsh continued. The Human Vaccines Project has developed its data policies with input from individuals who have experience with data hosting and sharing in order to create comprehensive data standards. The ethos is not to reinvent the wheel, but "to make sure all the wheels get on to one car so the car can move," she said.

Overview of the Model's Scientific Approach

The Human Vaccines Project's main strategic initiative is the creation of an environment that facilitates the planning and implementation of iterative clinical trials to speed up and expand the scale of what those clinical trials can do, said Welsh. The Human Vaccines Project's scientific approach focuses on key populations who are most at risk of developing disease. The project uses licensed and experimental vaccines as probes in clinical trials to address specific scientific questions, such as how the immune system develops specific responses, the durability of desired responses, how to identify the correlates of protection, and why some people respond while others do not.

The Human Vaccines Project's systems analyses include imprinting, transcriptomics, metabolomics, genomics, epigenomics, microbiomes, immunome, cytokine assays, antibody repertoire, flow cytometry, and controlled human challenge studies. Within clinical trials, the Human Vaccines Project performs immune profiling that is among the most comprehensive and in-depth ever performed, she said. Its network has the expertise to conduct antibody repertoire sequencing and immune system imprinting. It is working with lymph node fine-needle aspirates and bone marrow biopsies to look at germinal center responses, as well as multi-omic profiling to provide a holistic view of what is happening in the immune system before and after vaccination. Once the data are collected, the Human Vaccines Project's bioinformaticists work with specialists to integrate the data and present it in a clear and effective way.

In addition to conducting clinical trials, the Human Vaccines Project aims to leverage existing datasets and stored sample collections. She added that they have received approval from the Clinical Study Data Request Repository, which is a collection of sponsors who deposit clinical data in a repository that can be used for analyses.

Welsh explained that the Human Vaccines Project's ultimate goal is an AI-driven model of the immune system. By coupling AI with bioinformatics, the Human Vaccines Project hopes to make sense of the exponential leaps in the scale of data being generated—it is estimated that 1 trillion terabytes (1 yottabyte) of data would provide a complete picture of human biology per individual, she said. AI and machine learning will be central for the analysis of "big data" and will transform the future of vaccination, diagnostic, and therapeutic development, she added.

Another long-term goal for the Human Vaccines Project is to be able to run a clinical trial simulation based on real immunoresponse data. They intend to collect large amounts of immunoresponse data and run a simulation to see how a clinical trial candidate would do in the real world. This kind of simulation would enable initial testing of candidates that would allow developers to modify their candidates before clinical trials. She noted that in the early 2000s, the Human Genome Project engaged multiple sectors and countries to develop fundamental knowledge of genetics and the genetic blueprint. The Human Vaccines Project aims to do for immunology what the Human Genome Project did for genetics, by providing better understanding of the complex interactions that govern immune responses. Partnership across the board is needed in order to tackle these complex problems by collecting, analyzing, and presenting data in a way that is useful for the field, she said.

REVERSE INNOVATION

Maurizio Vecchione discussed the concept of reverse innovation as a radical approach to forging public–private partnerships and developing ecosystems of innovation to counter microbial threats. He explained that Global Good is a sister organization to the Bill & Melinda Gates Foundation, established to address global health priorities by conducting work through the Gates ecosystem of laboratories, scientists, and institutes. Given the opportunity costs and risks inherent in research and development, this work could not be conducted simply by granting funds to an institute.

He explained that because Global Good has virtually unlimited funding from a generous private donor, they are able to take risks that other entities cannot take. To leverage this advantage, Global Good's infrastructure is designed to absorb its investment and direct it to the riskiest parts of the world. Once the risk of a project is reduced, conventional partners take over the execution. In this way, Global Good's engagement model is to take on the greatest risks and support scale-up components, while leaving its partners with the lower risk.

Enabling Convergent Technologies to Address the Research and Development Gap

Vecchione discussed the implications of Global Good's work from a global ecosystem perspective. According to data from the 2017 Global Burden of Disease Study,[2] noncommunicable diseases account for 61 percent of deaths worldwide, with communicable diseases accounting for 28 percent and injuries accounting for 11 percent. Global datasets like these

[2] Data from the Global Burden of Disease Study are available from http://www.healthdata.org/gbd (accessed February 9, 2020).

may give the impression that the worldwide burden of communicable diseases is diminishing, he noted. However, this picture is misleading in that the Global Burden of Disease Study data are presented as a blended average for the entire world. Consequently, data from two countries—China and India—dominate the Global Burden of Disease Study. For the richest billion and poorest billion people, the burdens of disease are very different than the blended average burdens.

For the richest billion, noncommunicable diseases represent the majority of the burden of disease; for the poorest billion, communicable diseases account for more than half of the burden of disease. If divided into quartiles by daily income, the two lower quartiles of the global population have a far greater burden of communicable disease than the two higher quartiles. The human population is expected to reach 11 billion in the near future, he noted, at which point the majority of the population growth will occur in the two lower quartiles by daily income, meaning that communicable diseases will be substantial global threats.

Vecchione said that cancer and other noncommunicable diseases are important research priorities. However, in terms of global investment in research and development, a large gap exists in spending to address the burden of communicable diseases that affects the majority of the global population. Data from Booz & Co. in 2011 estimated annual investment in scientific research and development to be $600 billion, with health care research and development accounting for $130 billion. Only $3 billion is spent each year on research and development for G-FINDER's[3] 34 neglected diseases, including $2.1 billion on HIV, tuberculosis, and malaria (Moran et al., 2012). To address this gap in funding, the Bill & Melinda Gates Foundation and Global Good are addressing the "Great R&D Gap" by focusing on the diseases with the greatest impact on the bottom two quartiles of the global population by daily income.

Vecchione pointed out that there are multiple scientific revolutions under way that are enabling a variety of multidisciplinary and converging approaches to solving global health challenges. The methodologies for developing drugs, vaccines, and diagnostic tools are being transformed by new tools, such as AI. The development of next-generation AI is making strides toward making this true cognitive intelligence a reality that can be leveraged to address these challenges in the future. He explained that much of Global Good's work is designed to take a systemic approach to these threats, because it is not sufficient to focus on individual diseases, such as polio, in a siloed way that is centered on surveillance. Rather, it is necessary to strengthen health systems as a whole to make transitions into

[3] More information on the G-FINDER project can be found at https://www.policycuresresearch.org/g-finder (accessed March 30, 2020).

novel approaches to patient-centered treatment. Health care needs to be reinvented, because half of the 5 million children who will die in 2020 will die in the first 28 days of their lives (Goalkeepers, 2016).

Leapfrog Innovations and Transforming Data-Driven Technologies

Global Good focuses on reverse innovation because countries with nonexistent or poorly functioning health systems are prime groups for leapfrogging and innovating, said Vecchione. To illustrate, he described a leapfrog innovation in Kenya that uses mobile technology. Kenya has the highest use of mobile phones and the highest use of advanced data systems for mobile payment systems in the world. Because the country has no wire-line infrastructure or banking system, they leapfrogged and invented a banking system on mobile platforms, he noted.

Global Good's vision is to transform data-driven technologies to allow the technologies of the future to be designed and optimized in silico using computer models before they are ever manufactured, said Vecchione. Existing technologies already allow for modeling to predict the effect of an intervention on a disease before it is implemented. However, he noted that the real power of these models is not just in visualizing the situation as it exists today; the greater value comes from looking at potential future scenarios to understand what mix of resources is needed to improve the chances of eradication. For instance, Global Good is working on predicting the effectiveness of a particular set of parameter optimizations on a diagnostic for tuberculosis. Modeling suggests that the new test will have a significant effect on the number of new tuberculosis infections. This modeling is being done before ever building the diagnostic tools, he noted. This type of technology allows for the creation of the targets for intervention that will deliver patient-centered transformations in health care.

In Global Good's laboratory environment, teams are also creating the capacity to allow for the rapid development of new technology. For example, they have designed an AI-based robotic system that is tied to the epidemiological simulations and allows for the direct, automatic identification and optimization of new assays in record time. It takes Global Good approximately 6 months to develop a concept into a finished diagnostic product in the field with clinical trials, which collapses the normal development cycle for these types of technologies.

Vecchione presented an example of a project that used a multidisciplinary approach that leverages the traditional modality of ultrasound. By combining ultrasound with other technologies such as bioinformatics, Global Good developed the first portable automatic pneumonia assessment tool, which is being implemented into primary care in most countries in Africa. This new tool is 93 percent sensitive, 93 percent specific, and had 93 percent specificity in clinical trials, exceeding the sensitivity and specificity of X-rays with expert interpretation (Liu et al., 2013).

A similar breakthrough recently occurred in cervical cancer, he added. Because of the availability of a cervical cancer vaccine, cervical cancer is considered a solved problem—but this is only the case for those who can access the vaccine. Even if global access to the human papillomavirus (HPV) vaccine were achieved, an estimated 20 million more cases of cervical cancer will occur in the next 20 years before complete prevention of cervical cancer is realized (Gage and Castle, 2010). Global Good discovered that approximately 85 percent of cervical cancer deaths occur in low-resource settings because it has been difficult to establish the clinical laboratory infrastructure needed to conduct adequate screening via Pap smears. Global Good discovered that by using a blended approach, a simple camera phone picture of a woman's cervix could be used to predict cervical cancer more accurately than molecular histopathology or Pap smears through a specific kind of cognitive intelligence and machine learning (Hu et al., 2019). This approach has unlocked a new standard of care for women in 111 countries, he said. The technology was recently adopted by the World Health Assembly as the standard of care for cervical cancer screening in most of the world. Vecchione emphasized that this technology is an example of what can be achieved when a multidisciplinary approach is used to tie diagnostics to treatment and develop a system-level intervention that is patient centered and not siloed.

NURTURING INNOVATION TO ACCELERATE RESEARCH AND DEVELOPMENT

Sally Allain presented on nurturing innovation to accelerate research and development, using the example of Johnson & Johnson Innovation's model for driving external partnership, venture capital investment, and working across the entrepreneurial ecosystem. She explained that Johnson & Johnson is the largest and most diverse health care company in the world, working across three sectors: pharmaceuticals, consumer products, and medical devices and medical device innovation. The company has an internal mandate to innovate and an obligation to deliver innovative products to patients and consumers along with medicines that increase years of life, quality of life, and overall well-being.

Addressing Unique Needs of the Partnering Equation

The innovation level necessary for success has dramatically increased, said Allain. A product ought to be differentiated in order to be brought to market and surpass market expectations, so the company cannot rely on internal innovation alone. She said that Johnson & Johnson Innovation is agnostic in the way it innovates, with no preference for internal innovation over innovation through external partnership. Johnson & Johnson Innovation has a mutually beneficial relationship with external entrepreneurs, she explained. The company benefits from the innovation, small nimble teams, and cost savings that entrepreneurs bring, while entrepreneurs benefit from the capital, infrastructure, and expertise in development and commercialization that Johnson & Johnson Innovation can provide.

Allain described how Johnson & Johnson Innovation has developed comprehensive solutions to address unique needs of the partnering equation. When Johnson & Johnson Innovation began building a model for external innovation, it decided to embed itself into existing ecosystems using its network of innovation centers, its corporate venture arm Johnson & Johnson Development Corporation (JJDC), the JLABS Life Science Incubator model, and business development support. Together, these solutions make up Johnson & Johnson Innovation's comprehensive global solution for engagement with innovators across the consumer, health technology, medical devices, vision care, and pharmaceutical sectors. It offers entrepreneurs a "partner for every stage" by providing opportunities all along the research and development pipeline, from start-up and innovation to proof of concept, sector onboarding, and going to market. The JLABS model provides incubation and mentoring, while the innovation centers offer advice and mentorship, innovation acceleration, and research and development collaboration. Through their business development and strategic investment arms, it can provide equity investment and venture funding, strategic collaborations, licensing, acquisitions and divestments, and new company creations.

Innovation Centers

Four innovation centers are located in life science hotspots on three continents, with broad networks across regions connecting innovation ecosystems to the central innovation center hubs to create flexible collaborations, said Allain. The innovation centers focus on early-stage acceleration in the pipeline from discovery through early clinical studies; they house experts in pharmaceuticals, medical device innovation, and consumer products. She reported that the centers have facilitated more than 400 deals and deployed more than $1 billion since 2013.

Strategic Investment and Business Development Support

Strategic investors from JJDC offer extensive health care investing experience and work in partnership with the innovation centers to form new companies, said Allain. Mid- and late-stage business development deals are supported by business development teams from Janssen, Johnson & Johnson

Medical Devices and Johnson & Johnson Consumer, which provide help in licensing, mergers and acquisitions, and alliance management. Janssen Business Development works with established biotech and pharmaceutical companies at all stages of licensing and mergers and acquisitions.

JLABS Life Science Incubators

JLABS life science incubators create an enabling platform and an ecosystem that brings many groups together to drive innovations in science and technology in collaboration with entrepreneurs, said Allain. JLABS has 13 locations across the globe, including JPODS in North America, with 600 portfolio companies and more than 135 collaborations with Johnson & Johnson. JLABS engages across all sectors, including the consumer, health tech, medical device, and pharmaceutical sectors. She explained that JLABS offers the benefits of a large company's infrastructure to small companies.

Johnson & Johnson Innovation wants entrepreneurs to use its capital to drive their science and technology, which is why it offers access to centralized infrastructure, capital, equipment, benchtop facilities, and offices at low cost. It also provides educational programming to build skills, knowledge, and networks that empower and enable local innovation communities, along with funding series support to connect capital with innovators to increase the volume and velocity of deal flow. It creates cross-sector opportunities to build an environment for solutions and not only products, she added. Recognizing that companies are at various stages of development and may need different types of support, JLABS also offers mentorship and support ranging from preparation for clinical trials to medical device development to help move companies' products and drugs forward.

To promote open innovation and to help entrepreneurs build equity and value, JLABS uses a no-strings-attached model and does not ask for ownership of intellectual property. She noted that of the 23 JLABS portfolio companies that have gone public, 13 have been acquired, including a recent large acquisition of 1 portfolio company by Astellas for $3 billion. Around 88 percent of the JLABS portfolio companies are still in business or have been acquired, she added.

Collaboration with BARDA

Allain said that Johnson & Johnson Innovation partnered with BARDA in 2018. Through a specialized innovation zone, it provides residency for companies and entrepreneurs focused on solutions with the potential to improve the country's response, capacity, and capabilities to address evolving 21st-century health security threats. BARDA and JLABS will leverage their mutual expertise and resources to develop programs and initiatives that catalyze a new community of entrepreneurs, investors, and thought leaders committed to meeting the national medical defense needs by mounting a rapid and effective response against threats with innovative, end-to-end solutions.

One of the collaborations between BARDA and JLABS is the Invisible Shield QuickFire Challenge. For example, the current program invites action against airborne viruses, both in repelling and protecting against them, that could be easily integrated into daily life. Awardees receive grant funding, access to the JLABS ecosystem, and mentorship from expertise in the Johnson & Johnson family of companies. The first QuickFire challenge was awarded in October 2019 to Air99, which created a product that reimagines respiratory protection and air mask filters.

Allain described the progress of two companies that emerged from the JLAB portfolio. Inflammatix, Inc., is developing rapid diagnostics to distinguish between bacterial and viral infections and judge their severity, through gene expression patterns. BARDA will support the advanced development of the novel testing technology developed by Inflammatix. She also highlighted the collaboration between Janssen Pharmaceuticals and Locus Biosciences, who have signed an exclusive collaboration and license agreement for CRISPR[4] products intended to treat bacterial infections. The partners will develop and commercialize a CRISPR-Cas3-enhance bacteriophage candidate that targets two bacterial pathogens.

SPURRING INNOVATION IN DIAGNOSTIC TOOLS

Ranga Sampath emphasized that without appropriate diagnostic tools, the world's most pressing public health needs cannot be sustainably addressed because "without diagnosis, medicine is blind." For patients, diagnostics enable correct treatment and universal health coverage; for communities, diagnostics help halt the spread of antimicrobial resistance and disease outbreaks. For governments, diagnostics accelerate disease elimination, provide data for health interventions, and reduce spending. He remarked that despite the progress made over the past decades, the global community remains unprepared to grapple with an unknown virus or pathogen. His presentation focused on challenges and opportunities in improving diagnostics.

Foundation for Innovative New Diagnostics

Sampath explained that FIND was established in 2003 as a global nonprofit driving diagnostic innovation to combat major diseases affecting the world's poorest populations. FIND's business model is intended to address

[4] CRISPR is clustered regularly interspaced short palindromic repeats, a segment of DNA found in the genomes of prokaryotes.

areas of market failure by partnering to develop and deliver diagnostic solutions for low- and middle-income countries (LMICs). FIND is headquartered in Geneva with offices throughout Southeast Asia and Africa; it is interested in partnering with industries in Europe, Asia, North America, and elsewhere. For instance, China, India, and African nations have increasingly been moving toward models of in-country innovation, research, and design, so FIND intends to facilitate this trend by situating in-country efforts at the center of its work in advancing diagnostics.

FIND's areas of focus include antimicrobial resistance, hepatitis C, HIV, malaria, fever, neglected tropical diseases, pandemic preparedness, and tuberculosis. He noted that many of the challenges facing LMICs are driven by practices of the Global North, such as antibiotic dumping. FIND is a member of WHO's Strategic Advisory Group of Experts on In Vitro Diagnostics. This group offers a quality management system for in vitro diagnostics clinical trials certified by the International Organization for Standardization. Sampath said that FIND's business model has been successful in transforming tuberculosis diagnostics in LMICs using modern molecular technologies, and it is now seeking to expand those efforts across multiple diseases. FIND works openly and transparently across the industry with multiple partners, serving as a bridge between industry and WHO. Additionally, FIND is a diagnostic collaborating center and a laboratory strengthening partner at WHO. Diagnostics often require constant advocacy, which is also a routine part of FIND's activities.

Strategies for Delivering Effective Innovations

Sampath described the strategic pillars that FIND uses to tackle three "valleys of death" that need to be overcome in order to deliver effective new diagnostic tools to those who need them. High rates of attrition occur at each step in the evolution from concept to product development to commercialization to rollout of a diagnostic product. FIND works to address scientific, market, and policy failures and bridge the valleys of death between each of those stages in the process. To move from conceptualization and product development—the first valley—tools must be fit for the purpose and meet both countries' and patients' needs. FIND works in this space by catalyzing development.

The next valley—between product development and commercialization—is caused by the need for large data packages for regulatory and policy change. FIND addresses this valley by guiding use and policy. The third valley lies between commercialization and rollout, because multistakeholder engagement is required for financing, procurement, and workforce training. Sampath remarked that FIND works in this area by accelerating access. In addition to those three areas of activity, FIND works to shape the agenda through advocacy and publications to engage with funders and donors to support innovations.

To catalyze development by spurring diagnostic innovation across the value chain, FIND's partnership model is to work with developers of any size to ensure they are developing products that are the right solution for the right setting, said Sampath. In addition to bringing donor funding to developers, it also offers technical expertise, guidance, sample banking, data sharing, matchmaking, and other tools to enable its partners' success. FIND works across many technologies, from paper-based rapid diagnostic tests to complex molecular diagnostics.

Sampath provided examples of some of the projects that FIND is currently supporting, noting that FIND works agnostically across different technologies. Multiplex rapid diagnostic tests are being developed that can differentiate multiple causes of fever. Lab-in-a-box innovations can facilitate portable rapid assessment of pathogens with pandemic potential, while point-of-care molecular platforms can support confirmatory diagnosis at patients' bedsides. A next-generation sequencing solution for rapid assessment of drug-resistant tuberculosis pathogens across Brazil, China, India, Russia, and South Africa is also being developed, he said.

To demonstrate how FIND's co-investment model addresses market failure in LMICs, Sampath described some of their achievements. Between 2015 and 2018, FIND brought forward 16 new tools through its collaborative partnership model, in which companies bring in technology along with some type of in-kind or financial support. To guide use and policy, FIND has been instrumental in the development of 11 WHO recommendations, 71 clinical trials, and 32,500 patient enrollments. To accelerate access, FIND has helped train more than 6,000 health workers, strengthened more than 3,000 laboratories and sites, and provided more than 50 million FIND-supported products to recipients in 150 LMICs. FIND has shaped the agenda through the publication of 241 scientific articles.

The global health context is challenging and complex, said Sampath, so development must address country needs across the ecosystem to promote uptake. FIND partners with countries to address their downstream needs. He noted that it is important to ensure that pull from the country exists for a product, because sustainability is contingent on the country's demand, which can be quashed by donor funding. Considerations in these efforts include

- Policy and regulatory guidance,
- Training and advocacy,
- Capacity assessment and workforce preparation,
- Supporting local research and development,
- Establishing research and developing partnerships,
- Ensuring relevant local test menus,
- Promoting sustainable business models, and
- Conducting analytical and clinical validation.

Examples of Innovations Implemented in Countries

Sampath provided several examples of innovations that have been implemented in countries with support from FIND.

Paving the Way for Rapid Uptake

FIND helped to pave the way for rapid uptake of molecular tuberculosis point-of-care diagnostics in India, said Sampath. The country had been reliant on GeneXpert, which had to be imported and added costs that were a burden to local economies. Through partnership with FIND, India transitioned from GeneXpert testing to Truenat, a battery-operated, point-of-care testing device that is cheaper than GeneXpert and feeds data directly into Nikshay, India's tuberculosis elimination program. He added that India's tuberculosis program tendered almost 6 million of these tests in just 1 year, which illustrates how locally built technology can facilitate uptake of innovations.

Informing Antimicrobial Resistance Policy and Practice

FIND has embarked on a large-scale project to inform antimicrobial resistance policy and practice through an antimicrobial resistance (AMR) Diagnostics Use Accelerator, an initiative designed to gather crucial evidence for an AMR policy and practice guidelines globally and locally through a study of 22,000 patients with acute febrile illness in 6 countries: Burkina Faso, Ghana, India, Myanmar, Nepal, and Uganda. Sampath explained that the program is intended to gather harmonized global and local evidence to develop a package of interventions at the primary health care level. This package will include point-of-care tests, clinical algorithms, patient flows, and training and communication tools. The program will use clinical outcomes and antibiotic prescriptions for impact assessment, he added. The unique study design with harmonized protocols enables evaluation at country and global levels. He explained that data gathered from this project are intended to inform WHO and in-country policy makers in developing new patient care algorithms. Ultimately, this project is about democratizing diagnostics and engaging closely with patients, he said.

Platform Approaches to Improve Surveillance and Preparedness

FIND uses innovative platform approaches to improve surveillance and preparedness, said Sampath. Diagnostics laboratories often have to deal with a large number of tools developed by different diagnostics developers—Sampath likened this to each mobile phone app requiring a separate phone. FIND is working to leverage existing technologies while also incorporating new assays by brokering partnerships between players who can develop assays on existing platforms. This creates a semi-open platform approach that allows for the incubation of ideas across companies to encourage synergizing across existing platforms and technology to reduce cost and increase efficiency, he said. The approach maximizes value for countries by offering a platform for sentinel and other testing during nonoutbreak periods; it drives economies of scale in manufacturing, supply, and regulation—thus mitigating manufacturer resistance to making assays for small markets—and it enables innovative business partnerships.

This platform helps to encourage sustainable investment in product development during peace time to reduce the reliance on panic investment in technologies during an outbreak, said Sampath. For example, more than 70 companies submitted product development plans for a near-patient Ebola diagnostic test over the course of the West Africa outbreak, but only 7 companies received WHO emergency use approval and 11 received emergency use authorization from FDA. None of these companies received approval through nonemergency FDA or WHO mechanisms. Most of these companies have since left the market, with repeat outbreaks highlighting the national and international manufacturing gaps for those Ebola diagnostic tests. Similarly, the majority of companies developing Zika products dropped out of the market as the epidemic waned alongside funding.

Co-Creation of Digital Tools to Expand Diagnostic Impact

FIND has also supported the co-creation of digital tools to expand diagnostic impact, including the use of network optimization and other models to deploy technological solutions. It takes advantage of connectivity and other means to measure how these technologies are being used. For instance, FIND has co-created digital tools to reduce the delay in tuberculosis diagnosis, said Sampath. These efforts helped empower health care staff to improve tuberculosis care in Myanmar and ensured that more patients entered into the treatment pathway. Digital innovation can also address issues of poor data availability and the limited use of data.

Toward Sustainable Ecosystem Evolution

Sampath closed with a discussion of sustainability and opportunities for ecosystem evolution. He described a scenario where tuberculosis and HIV care are delivered in separate settings; in such a scenario, an individual with HIV and tuberculosis has to go to two locations to receive care. Synergy needs to be developed to eliminate this inefficiency, he said. Although many simple solutions have been developed, implementing these solutions is a complex task, in part because of stakeholders who are entrenched in existing systems. Silos must be broken down and funding mechanisms should be redesigned to enable multiple diseases to be addressed with little or no additional resources, he said.

True partnerships should be country driven and use demand-driven technologies and broaden the donor base, Sampath continued. Because so much of this work has traditionally been donor driven, it calls into question whether innovative funding models will be able to drive technology uptake sustainably. However, he suggested that potential funding mechanisms can make use of structured, innovative financing, including priority review vouchers, advance market commitments, and volume guarantees. He added that global partnerships and innovation are the waves of the future for pushing this agenda forward to ensure that the diagnostic needs of all countries are met, not just LMICs.

DISCUSSION

Matt Zahn asked about opportunities to spread the burden from public laboratories to private laboratories with respect to diagnostic testing during an outbreak response. Sampath remarked that the challenge of shifting testing into private laboratories lies in obtaining the requisite accreditations and approvals. However, he suggested that this could be addressed through forging public–private partnerships and collaborating prior to an outbreak.

Eva Harris asked how Global Good's cervical cancer innovation would figure into countries' broader protocols for cervical cancer care, which are complicated by challenges related to vaccination timing, linkages to care after diagnosis, and conducting follow-up. Vecchione explained that work is under way by international agencies and funders to integrate this novel diagnostic with high predictive value into the continuum of cervical cancer prevention and treatment, which is particularly challenging in low-resource settings. However, if the disease can be detected before it becomes cancer, there are well-established treatment protocols and related technologies that have been developed and would allow for diagnosis and treatment during the same point-of-care session.

The aim of this new technology is to transition cervical cancer treatment from a surgical procedure conducted by a specialist toward a prevention-like treatment. He added that this new technology is not intended to be an alternative to population-level vaccination; rather, it is being developed as a solution to contribute to cervical cancer elimination before population-level immunity is reached. Given the lack of national-level efforts to expand HPV vaccination, Global Good is working to link diagnosis to treatment and establish a new protocol that collapses access to services to the base of the pyramid of health care.

Rajeev Venkayya asked what Global Good has learned about engaging communities around user-centered design, uptake, and adoption. Vecchione replied that Global Good began working on health technology by providing huge budgets to laboratories that developed products through an "accidental pipeline"—that is, a pipeline of solutions in search of a problem. In public health, there have been numerous cases where a new technological solution has been deployed that cannot be scaled up or does not address the realities of a problem on the ground. One reason for this is that these technologies tend to be invented in laboratories without a proper understanding of the problem at hand or of the context in which the new technology will be deployed. However, most public health problems are not technology problems; they are systemic and multifaceted problems. He explained that Global Good adjusted by adopting the practice of understanding the problem first, before developing solutions.

Global Good has also made large investments in bioinformatics and data, which allow for the prediction of pathogen outbreaks at a district level anywhere in the world. They can also account for the effects of climate change on pathogenicity of some targets owing to genetic pressures of those pathogens. By combining data and evidence with human-centered design components, Global Good works to curate a list of problems and determine which problems require a technical solution that the organization can support.

Keiji Fukuda remarked that innovation is evolving at a rate that countries and communities cannot maintain without support from stakeholders; bringing in AI and machine learning will likely lead to even more rapid changes. Vecchione replied that the Bill & Melinda Gates Foundation tries to address gaps by reimagining problems through a lens of new technologies that may not be immediately endorsed by experts in the field. For example, when Global Good began working to address cervical cancer, leaders in the field said that machine learning could not work. He said that innovators must not let past failures inhibit them when striving to develop and iterate disruptive technologies. He added that governments, corporations, and donor-funded organizations have different levels of appropriate risk.

From a business perspective, innovators assume great risk because the odds of failure are high, and a certain degree of failure is to be expected. In business and government ecosystems, there is an aversion to this risk, which is why partnership with large-scale donors can foster innovation. It is donors' tolerance for risk that enables many innovations, including the cervical cancer innovation, which would not have been possible without donor-funded risk reduction of the technology. Vecchione encouraged innovators to keep this stratification of risk in mind as they pursue innovation; even within the Gates ecosystem, there are different tolerances for risk among different programs.

Sampath remarked that many of the technologies that are driving innovation were not developed based on a blueprint for how technology should solve health care problems; instead, they were successfully developed for other purposes and are now serving as a platform for innovative health care technology—such as mobile phones and communication technology. These technologies advance in leaps and bounds and thus will sometimes fail, but if the right questions are asked, then the right applications will usually be brought to bear. Often the challenge lies in asking the right questions and developing systemic answers to these questions, he added.

Allain commented that there are examples of simple innovations that can be developed relatively inexpensively by small companies with modest seed funding. For example, before Air99 innovated respiratory masks, the technology had not been changed for 50 years. Using a seed grant from Johnson & Johnson Innovation, Air99 developed a respiratory mask that would fit any type of face from infants to adults, which was an effective innovation that addressed a real need. Another company in the Johnson & Johnson Innovation portfolio is Certa Dose. It developed a color-coding system for syringes to reduce dosing errors, which has the potential to substantially improve the delivery of care, particularly in low-resource settings.

Welsh commented that investment firms can also mitigate risk. When the Human Vaccines Project began, it had financial partners who shared the risk of the project. The Human Vaccines Project's promise to these partners was that it would work in a different, more efficient way that could accommodate the needs of the research network, for example, by conducting flexible iterative clinical trials that begin with small groups then scale up depending on the needs of the product. These strategies allowed the Human Vaccines Project to change its risk profile for investors. The Human Vaccines Project provides smaller grants and other kinds of benefits—such as access to large datasets, immunology tools, and bioinformatics—that can support its partners in developing vaccines in a different way, which can offset the risk of investment.

Nitika Pant Pai asked about barriers and challenges that the Human Vaccines Project has faced in proposing a new method of immunology research. Welsh explained that it is challenging to sell the idea of the Human Vaccines Project, because donors perceive the project as similar to a think tank or innovation engine. Because the Human Vaccines Project is not a laboratory and is not developing a disease-specific vaccine, it is difficult for donors to understand the project. However, they are working to scale up and move from the pilot phase toward larger consortium-style projects. She suggested that once the Human Vaccines Project's infrastructure, data systems, and processes are in place, it will be easier to see the power of applying those data beyond research on infectious diseases and cancers.

Turkan Gardinier expressed concern about calling the outputs of research "intelligence." Systematic analysis and operations research have been widely used to find linkages between occurrences and the spread of diseases, but those analyses do not constitute intelligence. She cautioned against the use of language that suggests that these processes are developing intelligent systems that surpass human efforts. Vecchione replied that AI could more accurately be called "statistical intelligence," because machine learning reveals statistical correlations. He suggested that the exuberance about machine learning and the sentiment that it is the solution to all problems may be running its course.

Machine learning techniques work well in certain applications. However, they need to be blended with statistical stochastic models in many predictive models, especially when large populations and uncertainty across numerous factors are involved. He calls this blend "cognitive intelligence"—meaning, allowing a computer to become a thinking machine—and predicted that it will be the successor to AI. It is currently available in the average machine learning toolkit, he continued, but mechanistically driven forms of intelligence are being developed on the cutting edge of drug discovery. Although this technology is not yet practical to use, he suggested that it will revolutionize immunology and genome projects by extracting meaning from the correlations and distinguishing between causation and correlations.

George Haringhuizen asked about the potential for a global, well-curated sequence database of viruses and bacteria that could be used for day-to-day diagnostics. Sampath said that sequencing has great potential, but it is not a technological advancement that will solve the problem of diagnostics overall. Sequencing may be a piece of the solution in terms of content and processing ability, but technology cannot be a sole solution.

Vecchione commented that more technology is not necessarily better in terms of clinical care. He noted that there are more magnetic resonance imaging machines on the west side of Los Angeles than in all of western Europe combined; this does not mean that people in Los Angeles are healthier than people in western Europe. Sequencing is a tremendous revolutionary technology that will advance many areas of diagnostics, he said, but next-generation sequencing should be used to strengthen the patient-centered continuum of care. He also mentioned there are certain diagnostic innovations that cannot be relied on as a sole diagnostic tool because they do not address host–response mechanisms, comorbidity, or other factors that are addressed in the continuum of care. He suggested improving decision-making support along the clinical continuum of care so that the best diagnostic tools are being integrated into a system that is designed to facilitate the best treatment decisions.

Jyoti Joshi commented that technological innovation occurs so rapidly that it is difficult for clinicians, academics, or students to keep up with the evolving paradigm. She asked how all stakeholders can be better supported to avoid the fear of new technologies that was seen during the Ebola and Zika outbreaks, when vaccines were available, yet people were hesitant to get vaccinated.

Allain replied that when JLABS moves into an ecosystem where innovation is ongoing, it offers programming that addresses science, technology, venture capital, and business development for anyone who may wish to become involved. This is intended to foster open dialogue across stakeholders and reduce silos among them. The new JLABS site in Washington, DC, is located at the Children's National Hospital so innovators can work closely with the stakeholders whose problems they are innovating to address.

Vecchione remarked that in the near future, the bulk of the market for innovation will be outside of the United States, as countries like China and India accrue increasing spending power and capacity. He suggested that these emerging markets need to be empowered to enter into the ecosystem and innovate for themselves. This can be supported by building local capacity to incubate innovation and reverse innovation, he added. As an example, he described the "Silicon Savannah," an ecosystem of venture capital and entrepreneurs outside of Nairobi, Kenya, that is centered around mobile financial services. He suggested that existing, suboptimal practices that have been in use in Western countries are poised to be leapfrogged.

Welsh commented that there are different ways to disseminate information to catalyze young investigators to engage with these problems. For instance, the Human Vaccines Project oversees the Michelson Prize for young investigators who are interested in immunology. Such efforts not only spread the Human Vaccines Project's message and publicize its work, but they also encourage the next generation of scientists to innovate.

Marcos Espinal remarked that the most successful innovations seem to be shaped within partnerships that are focused on empowering and engaging with communities where the problems lie. For example, the Amazon Basin in Brazil has large burdens of malaria and dengue, but new technological innovations would not be appropriate for indigenous communities. In contrast, it would be beneficial for the country if the vaccines currently under development were manufactured in Brazil for its own people.

Vecchione pointed out that Global Good's work in cervical cancer encountered cultural issues that were not addressed by their technological innovations. For example, communities tended to mistrust government representatives, which undermined any implementation that relied on a government mandate to screen every woman in each community. To address this barrier, Global Good engaged with community health workers—typically older women—who evangelized for cervical cancer screening within their communities on behalf of the implementers of this program. This approach has not been scaled up, but it demonstrates the importance of stakeholder engagement, he noted.

8

Visionary Statements on Priorities for Innovation

The final part of the workshop's last session featured visionary statements. The three panelists were Julio Croda, chief, Department of Communicable Diseases, Secretary of Health Surveillance, Brazil; Lori Burrows, associate director, Michael G. DeGroote Institute for Infectious Disease Research, Canada; and Peter Sands, executive director, The Global Fund to Fight AIDS, Tuberculosis and Malaria (The Global Fund). Moderated by Marcos Espinal, director, Department of Communicable Diseases and Environmental Determinants of Health, Pan American Health Organization, the panelists synthesized priority actions on cultivating innovative solutions to address emerging microbial threats that are sustainable, ethical, equitable, and focused on interventions that most effectively improve people's lives.

INNOVATIONS AGAINST VECTOR-BORNE DISEASES IN BRAZIL

Julio Croda remarked that developing the simplest and cheapest innovations is the best strategy to ensure that solutions are feasible and can be implemented across settings with different resource levels. He provided several examples of health innovations being delivered to the poorest populations in Brazil. Two arbovirus control innovations are being planned to scale up across the country.

One project involves large-scale release of *Aedes aegypti* mosquitoes with *Wolbachia* bacteria in urban areas to assess their effect on dengue fever and other vector-borne diseases, such as chikungunya and Zika (van den Hurk et al., 2012). *Wolbachia* are inherited intracellular bacterial symbionts common in many mosquitoes, but not in mosquito species considered to be of major importance in transmitting human pathogens (Moreira et al., 2009). In Brazilian *Aedes aegypti* mosquitoes, *Wolbachia* has been found to block circulating Zika virus isolates (Dutra et al., 2016). Studies have also determined that this intervention reduces the transmission potential of dengue-infected *Aedes aegypti* (Ye et al., 2015). An ongoing clinical trial is looking at the effect of this intervention on the offspring of *Wolbachia*-infected and wild-type mosquitoes.

Another innovation, the Arbo-Alvo project, is a methodological proposal for risk stratification for dengue, chikungunya, and Zika in endemic cities in Brazil. Among the project's goals are to evaluate and identify areas of increased risk for dengue transmission using local spatial statistics in certain territories. When combined with other innovations, this package can be used to optimize control of the arbovirus. The SISS-Geo platform was created in 2014 to assist in monitoring the health of wildlife in Brazil, in collaboration with communities, health professionals, the environmental sector, and researchers, through mobile devices and a web platform. Based on information from the platform, mathematical modeling can be used to predict the number of human cases of yellow fever and inform vaccination efforts.

Another project is using single-dose tafenoquine combined with G6PD rapid testing to track malaria transmission in northern Brazil. To address visceral leishmaniasis, researchers are implementing more than 2 million insecticide-impregnated dog collars in the regions of Brazil heavily affected by the disease. Finally, he noted that a prison-based tuberculosis intervention is being implemented, because mathematical modeling suggests that exit screening is more effective than entry screening to detect the spread of the disease in prisons and to reduce the spillover effect in the general community (Mabud et al., 2019).

INNOVATIONS TO ADDRESS ANTIMICROBIAL RESISTANCE IN CANADA

Lori Burrows opened by citing a recent report by the Council of Canadian Academies, *When Antibiotics Fail* (CCA, 2019). She explained that although Canada has a strong health care system, it is somewhat fragmented because health care is delivered provincially, so each province has slightly different demographics, faces different problems, and monitors different indicators. This is a challenge for the development of national-level statistics, such as the number of people who actually die of drug-resistant infections, which was not available prior to this report. This illustrates why a problem needs to be clearly defined and quantified before government resources can be requested and deployed to address it, she noted.

To encourage government action, the report also clearly defines the socioeconomic cost of failing to address antimicrobial resistance (AMR) in Canada. As of December 2019, 26 percent of infections in the country are resistant to first-line antibiotics; this is likely to increase to 40 percent by 2030, stated Burrows. She suggested that the estimated $1.4 billion in health care costs and $2 billion in lost gross domestic product currently associated with AMR will also increase commensurately. Another benefit of the report is that it contains stories and vignettes of real people who have been affected by AMR, she said, and engaging people at a personal level can garner more resources for a problem. Current work to address AMR in Canada is being supported by private donors who acquired drug-resistant infections themselves, as the government is not yet willing to provide funding.

Burrows emphasized that regardless of the setting's resource level, dealing with drug-resistant infections requires cross-sector innovations in stewardship, surveillance, discovery, and economics. In the context of stewardship, she highlighted education as one of the keystones of addressing AMR. This should involve educating patients as well as physicians to decrease the prescription of unnecessary antibiotics, she said. Simply by training primary care physicians not to prescribe antibiotics for viral infections in children aged 0–14 years, the number of those prescriptions has decreased dramatically in that age group over the past decade in Canada, although similar decreases were not seen among healthy individuals middle aged or older (CCA, 2019). Cross-sectoral surveillance is required for monitoring pathogens and targeted deployment, she added. A recent World Bank report argued for building surveillance and management, integrated between human and veterinary medicine, in all countries, citing this as the most efficient and cost-effective solution to problems with antimicrobial resistance (Jonas et al., 2017).

In terms of economics, Burrows noted that new funding models and incentive models are needed. The pharmaceutical sector has divested itself significantly from antibiotic discovery given the risk of investing billions of dollars in developing drugs that could lose effectiveness owing to resistance within a short amount of time. She suggested that new ways to sell antibiotics are needed. For instance, an innovation is being piloted in Britain in a "Netflix-style" subscription model, whereby companies would develop antibiotics, and the hospitals and health care systems would pay into a subscription model in order to have access to those drugs if they need them. Another example is the nonprofit model used by Canadian Blood Services, which sends tenders out to companies to purchase large lots of factor VIII and factor IX, so that hospitals can directly request the products from Canadian Blood Services when they are needed, rather than requiring individual hospitals to procure the products themselves. She suggested that this existing infrastructure could be used to facilitate antibiotic stewardship, if the government were willing to do so.

Burrows stated that cross-sectoral innovations in discovery are already ongoing to develop new drugs, adjuvants, alternatives, vaccines, and diagnostics. She noted that in addition to being useful against viral diseases, vaccines are also useful against bacterial diseases and AMR (i.e., a person who is vaccinated against a bacterial disease and does not acquire the disease will not need to be treated with antibiotics). She works with *Pseudomonas aeruginosa* and *Acinetobacter baumannii*, gram-negative pathogens that are also opportunistic, which makes it challenging to determine whom to vaccinate, how often to vaccinate, and how to determine the efficacy of a potential vaccine. Bacteriophages represent a promising model for alternate ways to kill gram-negative drug-resistant pathogens. However, bacteriophages are not generally suitable for traditional clinical trials because they are so host specific—starting treatment with phages requires knowing the exact cause of a patient's infection.

Preserving bacteriophages is another multifactorial problem. Work is ongoing to find ways to preserve them on the shelf at room temperature for long periods of time so people in lower-resource countries can have access to them. She added that in addition to new antibiotics, new nutritional interventions are also needed. For example, urinary tract infections are one of the most common reasons why people are prescribed antibiotics in the community. Taking D-mannose can help prevent *Escherichia coli* urinary tract infections (Domenici et al., 2016), although this would be difficult to monetize. She noted that microbiome interventions hold promise in preventing infections, but the field is still nascent and hampered by pseudoscience. In terms of diagnostics, pairing inexpensive, paper-based diagnostics with interventions such as bacteriophages could represent alternate ways to treat infections in low-resource countries.

INNOVATIONS TO MAXIMIZE IMPACT IN AIDS, TUBERCULOSIS, AND MALARIA

Peter Sands explained that his organization is the largest multinational funding vehicle in global health, with an unprecedented $14 billion to spend through 2023. The Global Fund is not interested in innovation for innovation's sake, he said. They are interested in innovation if it can be scaled to "move the dial" and make a difference in the delivery of the organization's mandate to save lives and end the epidemics of HIV, tuberculosis, and malaria. As an organization, it has limited capacity to pursue innovations with interesting but marginal potential effects. In assessing innovations coming down the pipeline, The Global Fund focuses on the relative cost-effectiveness of new interventions versus expanding coverage of existing interventions, none of which are yet fully optimized. For instance, as a relatively cost-effective way to achieve greater effect, The Global Fund is looking for better ways to deploy condoms. Although they are inexpensive and highly effective when used well, they are currently poorly deployed and used, leading to substantial differences in their effectiveness across settings.

Another priority for The Global Fund is for innovation to be deeply informed by insights from the communities that are affected by those three diseases, said Sands. He also observed that innovations need to be scalable. Small pilot projects can showcase interesting new technologies, but The Global Fund is focused on interventions that can work at scale to change the lives of hundreds of thousands or millions of people. For example, ongoing work around self-testing for HIV is not widely integrated into national AIDS programs, leading to a large falloff from treatment among people who test positive within small pilot programs. The Global Fund will channel $25 million in catalytic funding toward integrating self-testing programs into national programs, which it has identified as the best way to effect real change, he added.

Sands explained that The Global Fund is seeking innovations that work within their time frames and within their model of country-informed decision making. Most of the organization's funding will be committed in signed grants for programs by the end of 2020, and the innovators with whom they work most successfully have a deep understanding of The Global Fund's mechanisms. He noted that progress moves slowly in the health world, for many good reasons, but suggested that there may be room for greater focus on the "time value of money" measured in lives (e.g., the lives lost due to lengthy delays in changing treatment guidelines for tuberculosis and HIV to incorporate new and improved regimens). He observed that there is an iteration in innovation between efforts to develop tools and then find uses for them, and efforts to identify problems and then find the tools to solve them. His organization is engaging people in the innovation sphere around HIV, tuberculosis, and malaria so they are aware of the problems of greatest concern and so The Global Fund has an idea of the tools that innovation could bring.

Sands remarked on the types of innovations that might interest The Global Fund in its three disease areas. In HIV, the immediate focus is on driving change in prevention: innovation is needed to help address why adolescent girls and younger women have much higher infection rates in many parts of Africa (Karim and Baxter, 2019). He noted that this may involve biomedical innovation, such as a combination contraceptive and preexposure prophylaxis regimen, as well as innovation around how to address gender-based violence. Additional scalable innovations are needed to break down human-rights-related barriers to accessing HIV care that are faced by people who are criminalized, marginalized, and stigmatized; people who are transgender; men who have sex with men; prisoners; and people who inject drugs, among many others.

Another issue warranting innovation is effectively engaging asymptomatic men with HIV with health systems, because these men are a major source of ongoing infection. Sands said that in the area of malaria, The Global Fund is involved in a pilot for a promising vaccine candidate. Sands noted that innovations are urgently needed around vector control that are inexpensive and cost-effective, because the average spend per capita in settings where malaria is highly endemic is only about $4 per year. In tuberculosis, he said that progress toward a vaccine is further out but still encouraging. In the shorter term, inexpensive robust diagnostics that do not require a laboratory-style environment, as well as better strategies to find people who have tuberculosis and determine whether the strain is drug sensitive, would be impactful.

FINAL SYNTHESIS AND DISCUSSION

Espinal asked how parallel, vertical innovations and initiatives like those supported by The Global Fund can parlay into health system strengthening, particularly in lower-income countries. Sands replied that there is no contradiction between having a mandate around the three biggest infectious diseases and supporting health system development, because countries that have been able to eliminate those diseases have done so by building strong health systems. In settings with high burdens of those three diseases, health systems tend to become overwhelmed and focus primarily on treating those diseases. He added that The Global Fund is the largest multinational investor in health systems, investing about $1 billion each year (Sands, 2018).

Innovation is also needed around health systems and particularly around community health worker models, on which the most resource-poor countries are dependent. Finding ways to use technology to support community health workers could help reduce their paperwork burden. He said that innovation in financing models would benefit countries with large informal economies where traditional tax or insurance modes of financing health do not work well. Croda highlighted the need to incorporate innovation in resource-poor countries without strong health systems by engaging policy makers to invest in innovation. Burrows commented that climate change needs to figure into these conversations, because many of the issues being discussed, such as migration and disease transmission, are the consequence of inequalities caused by climate change.

Rafael Obregón remarked that governments often lack the resources and capacity to evaluate the range of innovations and technologies available. He asked about how to support governments in deciding which innovations to move forward with, such as by helping to streamline decision-making processes. Sands responded that one strategy is for countries to channel their assistance on the three major infectious diseases through The Global Fund, which lessens the coordination costs of multiple different actors and provides a model by which the decision making is located in-country through the country coordinating mechanism. In settings where this strategy is feasible, working with local systems (e.g., government malaria agencies) is effective in addressing the diseases and building local capacities simultaneously, he said.

Audrey Lenhart asked about the level of evidence that would be sufficient to justify scaling up innovative interventions nationwide, such as the *Wolbachia* intervention in Brazil or the malaria vector control interventions supported by The Global Fund. Croda replied that the *Wolbachia* intervention will be supported by evidence from the ongoing phase 3 study. Governments are interested in a business plan to support these types of new innovations, he added. In HIV, for example, introducing a new drug and documenting how it has controlled transmission and reduced incidence can be used to inform the business plan to encourage governments to scale up the innovation.

Sands commented that in the context of next-generation bed nets for malaria, scale up of the pilot programs is currently constrained by manufacturing capacity. When that issue is resolved, the focus will be on deciding whether there is enough evidence to start scaling up in areas with the most prima facie evidence of vector resistance to the existing pyrethrum-based insecticides. This involves a complicated mix of scientific considerations about evidence-based decision making and ethical considerations—such as whether the interventions should be used in settings where the existing nets are not working as well—and communication issues. If confidence in the existing nets is undermined prematurely, then large numbers of existing nets might go unused. He added that stratification is another consideration. Understanding where resistance is located can ensure that those settings are targeted with the new nets, which are more expensive than the old nets. Sands concluded by highlighting the complicated trade-off between rolling out older nets to people who are not covered at all and upgrading the nets for those who are at the greatest risk.

References

Amman, B. R., S. A. Carroll, Z. D. Reed, T. K. Sealy, S. Balinandi, R. Swanepoel, A. Kemp, B. R. Erickson, J. A. Comer, S. Campbell, D. L. Cannon, M. L. Khristova, P. Atimnedi, C. D. Paddock, R. J. Crockett, T. D. Flietstra, K. L. Warfield, R. Unfer, E. Katongole-Mbidde, R. Downing, J. W. Tappero, S. R. Zaki, P. E. Rollin, T. G. Ksiazek, S. T. Nichol, and J. S. Towner. 2012. Seasonal pulses of Marburg virus circulation in juvenile *Rousettus aegyptiacus* bats coincide with periods of increased risk of human infection. *PLOS Pathogens* 8(10):e1002877.

Ansah, E. K., M. Gyapong, S. Narh-Bana, C. Bart-Plange, and C. J. Whitty. 2016. Factors influencing choice of care-seeking for acute fever comparing private chemical shops with health centres and hospitals in Ghana: A study using case-control methodology. *Malaria Journal* 15(1):290.

Bandyopadhyay, A. S. 2019. *Applying lessons learned from innovation in polio eradication.* PowerPoint presented at the workshop on Exploring the Frontiers of Innovation to Tackle Microbial Threats, Washington, DC.

Bandyopadhyay, A. S., J. Garon, K. Seib, and W. A. Orenstein. 2015. Polio vaccination: Past, present and future. *Future Microbiology* 10(5):791–808.

Bhatt, S., D. J. Weiss, E. Cameron, D. Bisanzio, B. Mappin, U. Dalrymple, K. E. Battle, C. L. Moyes, A. Henry, D. L. Smith, P. W. Gething, P. A. Eckhoff, E. A. Wenger, O. Briet, M. A. Penny, T. A. Smith, O. Briet, M. A. Penny, T. A. Smith, A. Bennett, J. Yukich, T. P. Eisele, J. T. Griffin, C. A. Fergus, M. Lynch, R. E. Cibulskis, F. Lindgren, J. M. Cohen, C. L. J. Murray, D. L. Smith, S. I. Hay, D. L. Smith, D. L. Smith, S. I. Hay, and S. I. Hay. 2015. The effect of malaria control on *Plasmodium falciparum* in Africa between 2000 and 2015. *Nature* 526(7572):207–211.

Bill & Melinda Gates Foundation. n.d. *Polio.* https://www.gatesfoundation.org/what-we-do/global-development/polio (accessed March 3, 2020).

Buckee, C. O., M. I. E. Cardenas, J. Corpuz, A. Ghosh, F. Haque, J. Karim, A. S. Mahmud, R. J. Maude, K. Mensah, N. V. Motaze, M. Nabaggala, C. J. E. Metcalf, S. A. Mioramalala, F. Mubiru, C. M. Peak, S. Pramanik, J. M. Rakotondramanga, E. Remera, I. Sinha, S. Sovannaroth, A. J. Tatem, and W. Zaw. 2018. Productive disruption: Opportunities and challenges for innovation in infectious disease surveillance. *BMJ Global Health* 3(1):e000538.

CCA (Council of Canadian Academies). 2019. *When Antibiotics Fail.* Ottawa, ON, Canada: The Expert Panel on the Potential Socio-Economic Impacts of Antimicrobial Resistance in Canada, Council of Canadian Academies.

CDC (U.S. Centers for Disease Control and Prevention). 2018. *Deadly Marburg virus found in Sierra Leone bats.* https://www.cdc.gov/media/releases/2018/p1220-marburg-found-in-bats.html (accessed February 18, 2020).

CDC. 2019a. *Ebola (Ebola Virus Disease): Signs and symptoms.* https://www.cdc.gov/vhf/ebola/symptoms/index.html (accessed March 3, 2020).

CDC. 2019b. *Years of Ebola virus disease outbreaks.* https://www.cdc.gov/vhf/ebola/history/chronology.html?CDC_AA_refVal=https%3A%2F%2Fwww.cdc.gov%2Fvhf%2Febola%2Foutbreaks%2Fhistory%2Fchronology.html (accessed March 4, 2020).

CDC. 2019c. *Preparedness pays off with quick response time.* https://www.cdc.gov/globalhealth/stories/ebola-preparedness.html (accessed March 4, 2020).

CDC. 2020. *One Health.* https://www.cdc.gov/onehealth/index.html (accessed March 26, 2020).

Chang, H. H., A. Mahmud, R. J. Maude, C. Buckee, H. H. Chang, A. Mahmud, R. J. Maude, C. Buckee, A. Wesolowski, I. Sinha, D. Uddin, S. I. Zaman, M. A. Faiz, M. Dhorda, O. Miotto, R. J. Maude, I. Sinha, M. Dhorda, R. J. Maude, C. G. Jacob, E. Drury, S. Goncalves, M. Kekre, O. Miotto, D. Kwiatkowski, M. A. Hossain, M. A. Faiz, A. Ghose, A. A. Sayeed, M. R. Rahman, A. Islam, M. J. Karim, M. M. Aktaruzzaman, M. K. Rezwan, A. K. M. Shamsuzzaman, S. T. Jhora, M. Dhorda, R. Vongpromek, O. Miotto, D. Kwiatkowski, and K. Engo-Monsen. 2019. Mapping imported malaria in Bangladesh using parasite genetic and human mobility data. *eLife* 8.

Cheng, M., R. Satter, and J. Goodman. 2016. Few Zika samples are being shared by Brazil, worrying international researchers. *Associated Press*, February 3, 2016.

Cima, G. 2020. Pandemic prevention program ending after 10 years: USAID PREDICT led virus discovery, health training, risk education. *Journal of the American Veterinary Medical Association News.* https://www.avma.org/javma-news/2020-01-15/pandemic-prevention-program-ending-after-10-years (accessed March 5, 2020).

Cochi, S. L., and W. R. Dowdle. 2013. *Disease eradication in the 21st century: Implications for global health.* Cambridge, MA: The MIT Press.

Crozier, I. 2016. Ebola virus rna in the semen of male survivors of Ebola virus disease: The uncertain gravitas of a privileged persistence. *Journal of Infectious Diseases* 214(10):1467–1469.

DFID (Department for International Development). 2019. UK aid to help vaccinate more than 400 million children a year against polio. https://www.gov.uk/government/news/uk-aid-to-help-vaccinate-more-than-400-million-children-a-year-against-polio (accessed March 4, 2020).

Diallo, B., D. Sissoko, N. J. Loman, H. A. Bah, H. Bah, M. C. Worrell, L. S. Conde, R. Sacko, S. Mesfin, A. Loua, J. K. Kalonda, N. A. Erondu, B. A. Dahl, S. Handrick, I. Goodfellow, L. W. Meredith, M. Cotten, U. Jah, R. E. Guetiya Wadoum, P. Rollin, N. Magassouba, D. Malvy, X. Anglaret, M. W. Carroll, R. B. Aylward, M. H. Djingarey, A. Diarra, P. Formenty, S. Keôta, S. Günther, A. Rambaut, and S. Duraffour. 2016. Resurgence of Ebola virus disease in Guinea linked to a survivor with virus persistence in seminal fluid for more than 500 days. *Clinical Infectious Diseases* 63(10):1353–1356.

Domenici, L., M. Monti, C. Bracchi, M. Giorgini, V. Colagiovanni, L. Muzii, and P. Benedetti Panici. 2016. D-mannose: A promising support for acute urinary tract infections in women. A pilot study. *European Review for Medical and Pharmacological Science* 20(13):2920–2925.

Dosani, R. F. 2019. *Fostering new partnerships to enable innovation.* PowerPoint presented at the workshop on Exploring the Frontiers of Innovation to Tackle Microbial Threats, Washington, DC.

Dusfour, I., J. Vontas, J., David, D. Weetman, D. M. Fonseca, V. Corbel, K. Raghavendra, M. B. Coullibaly, A. J. Martins, S. Kasai, and F. Chandre. 2019. Management of insecticide resistance in the major *Aedes* vectors of arboviruses: Advances and challenges. *PLOS Neglected Tropical Diseases* 13(10):e0007615.

Dutra, H. L., M. N. Rocha, F. B. Dias, S. B. Mansur, E. P. Caragata, and L. A. Moreira. 2016. *Wolbachia* blocks currently circulating Zika virus isolates in Brazilian *Aedes Aegypti* mosquitoes. *Cell Host and Microbe* 19(6):771–774.

Dzau, V. J., G. S. Ginsburg, A. Chopra, D. Goldman, E. D. Green, D. G. B. Leonard, M. McClellan, A. Plump, S. F. Terry, and K. R. Yamamoto. 2016. Realizing the full potential of precision medicine in health and health care: A vital direction for health and health care. *NAM Perspectives.* Discussion Paper, National Academy of Medicine, Washington, DC. https://doi.org/10.31478/201609k.

FDA (U.S. Food and Drug Administration). 2014. *First rapid home-use HIV kit approved for self-testing.* https://www.fda.gov/consumers/consumer-updates/first-rapid-home-use-hiv-kit-approved-self-testing (accessed March 4, 2020).

Forbes, K. M., P. W. Webala, A. J. Jaaskelainen, S. Abdurahman, J. Ogola, M. M. Masika, I. Kivisto, H. Alburkat, I. Plyusnin, L. Levanov, E. M. Korhonen, E. Huhtamo, D. Mwaengo, T. Smura, A. Mirazimi, O. Anzala, O. Vapalahti, and T. Sironen. 2019. Bombali virus in *Mops condylurus* bat, Kenya. *Emerging Infectious Diseases* 25(5).

Freudenthal, E. 2019. Ebola's lost blood: Row over samples flown out of Africa as "big pharma" set to cash in. *The Telegraph*, February 6, 2019.

Frost, I., J. Craig, J. Joshi, K. Faure, and R. Laxminarayan. 2019. *Access barriers to antibiotics.* Washington, DC: Center for Disease Dynamics, Economics & Policy.

Gage, J. C., and P. E. Castle. 2010. Preventing cervical cancer globally by acting locally: If not now, when? *Journal of the National Cancer Institute* 102(20):1524–1527.

Gandra, S., J. Joshi, A. Trett, A. Sankhil Lamkang, and R. Laxminarayan. 2017. Scoping report on antimicrobial resistance in India. Washington, DC: Center for Disease Dynamics, Economics & Policy.

Goalkeepers. 2016. *Case study: Child mortality.* https://datareport.goalkeepers.org/case-studies/child-mortality (accessed February 2, 2020).

Goldstein, T., B. H. Bird, A. Tremeau-Bravard, M. N. Belaganahalli, J. K. Dhanota, B. R. Smith, C. Monagin, C. K. Johnson, J. A. K. Mazet, S. J. Anthony, H. L. Wells, E. Liang, M. Grodus, W. I. Lipkin, S. J. Anthony, W. I. Lipkin, S. J. Anthony, E. Liang, A. Gbakima, J. Bangura, R. K. Jangra, V. A. DeJesus, K. Chandran, G. Lasso, S. Shapira, A. Jambai, B. O. Kamara, S. Kamara, W. Bangura, C. Monagin, K. Saylors, E. M. Rubin, and S. Shapira. 2018. The discovery of Bombali virus adds further support for bats as hosts of Ebola viruses. *Nature Microbiology* 3(10):1084–1089.

Grayson, K. 2016. Cultivating trust is critical—and surprisingly complex. *Kellogg Insight.* https://insight.kellogg.northwestern.edu/article/cultivating-trust-is-critical-and-surprisingly-complex (accessed March 4, 2020).

Hallsworth, M., T. Chadborn, A. Sallis, M. Sanders, D. Berry, F. Greaves, L. Clements, and S. C. Davies. 2016. Provision of social norm feedback to high prescribers of antibiotics in general practice: A pragmatic national randomised controlled trial. *The Lancet* 387(10029):1743–1752.

Haynes, K. E., and A. S. Fotheringham. 1984. *Gravity and spacial interaction models*. Beverly Hills, CA: Sage.

Hendriksen, R. S., P. Munk, P. Njage, B. van Bunnik, L. McNally, O. Lukjancenko, T. Roder, D. Nieuwenhuijse, S. K. Pedersen, J. Kjeldgaard, R. S. Kaas, P. Clausen, J. K. Vogt, P. Leekitcharoenphon, M. G. M. van de Schans, T. Zuidema, A. M. de Roda Husman, S. Rasmussen, B. Petersen, Global Sewage Surveillance Project Consortium, C. Amid, G. Cochrane, T. Sicheritz-Ponten, H. Schmitt, J. R. M. Alvarez, A. Aidara-Kane, S. J. Pamp, O. Lund, T. Hald, M. Woolhouse, M. P. Koopmans, H. Vigre, T. N. Petersen, and F. M. Aarestrup. 2019. Global monitoring of antimicrobial resistance based on metagenomics analyses of urban sewage. *Nature Communications* 10(1):1124.

Hu, L., D. Bell, S. Antani, Z. Xue, K. Yu, M. P. Horning, N. Gachuhi, B. Wilson, M. S. Jaiswal, B. Befano, L. R. Long, R. Herrero, M. H. Einstein, R. D. Burk, M. Demarco, J. C. Gage, A. C. Rodriguez, N. Wentzensen, and M. Schiffman. 2019. An observational study of deep learning and automated evaluation of cervical images for cancer screening. *Journal of the National Cancer Institute* 111(9):923–932.

Human Vaccines Project. 2020. *A new approach to fighting disease*. https://www.humanvaccinesproject.org (accessed March 5, 2020).

IVCC (Innovative Vector Control Consortium). n.d. *New Nets Project (NNP)*. https://www.ivcc.com/market-access/new-nets-project (accessed February 18, 2020).

Janssen, R., N. Engel, A. Esmail, S. Oelofse, A. Krumeich, K. Dheda, and N. P. Pai. 2020. Alone but supported: A qualitative study of an HIV self-testing app in an observational cohort study in South Africa. *AIDS and Behavior* 24(2):467–474.

Jonas, O. B., A. Irwin, F. C. J. Berthe, F. G. Le Gall, and P. V. Marquez. 2017. *Drug-resistant infections: A threat to our economic future*. Washington, DC: HNP/Agriculture Global Antimicrobial Resistance Initiative.

Jusu, M. O., G. Glauser, J. F. Seward, M. Bawoh, J. Tempel, M. Friend, D. Littlefield, M. Lahai, H. M. Jalloh, A. B. Sesay, A. F. Caulker, M. Samai, V. Thomas, N. Farrell, and M. A. Widdowson. 2018. Rapid establishment of a cold chain capacity of –60 degrees C or colder for the STRIVE Ebola vaccine trial during the Ebola outbreak in Sierra Leone. *Journal of Infectious Diseases* 217(Suppl 1):S48–S55.

Kahn, R., A. S. Mahmud, A. Schroeder, L. H. Aguilar Ramirez, J. Crowley, J. Chan, and C. O. Buckee. 2019. Rapid forecasting of cholera risk in Mozambique: Translational challenges and opportunities. *Prehospital and Disaster Medicine* 34(5):557–562.

Kahneman, D. 2003. A perspective on judgment and choice: Mapping bounded rationality. *American Psychologist* 58(9):697.

Karim, S. S. A., and C. Baxter. 2019. HIV incidence rates in adolescent girls and young women in sub-Saharan Africa. *Lancet Global Health* 7(11):e1470–e1471.

Keegan, S. 2014. Kiss of death: Defiant farmers still smooching camels despite deadly virus warnings. *Mirror*, May 14, 2014.

Kim, W. 2019. *Sparking antibiotic discovery through data sharing and scientific collaboration*. PowerPoint presented at the workshop on Exploring the Frontiers of Innovation to Tackle Microbial Threats, Washington, DC.

Koopmans, M., X. de Lamballerie, T. Jaenisch, K. D. Rosenberger, I. Morales, E. T. A. Marques, I. F. T. Viana, P. Brasil, R. Rabello, V. I. Avelino-Silva, A. Segurado, N. Alexander, P. Mayaud, E. M. Netto, A. Tami, S. Bethencourt, M. Consuelo Miranda, A. Lozano, C. Soria, S. P. Salgado Cisneros, E. Gotuzzo, M. G. Guzmán, P. A. M. Rodriguez, H. Lopez-Gatell, J. Hegewisch-Taylor, V. H. Borja-Aburto, C. Gonzales Bonilla, B. Hoen, M. van Roode, and B. Rockx. 2019. Familiar barriers still unresolved—A perspective on the Zika virus outbreak research response. *The Lancet Infectious Diseases* 19(2):e59–e62.

Kruk, M. E., A. D. Gage, C. Arsenault, K. Jordan, H. H. Leslie, S. Roder-DeWan, O. Adeyi, P. Barker, B. Daelmans, S. V. Doubova, M. English, E. G. Elorrio, F. Guanais, O. Gureje, L. R. Hirschhorn, L. Jiang, E. Kelley, E. T. Lemango, J. Liljestrand, A. Malata, T. Marchant, M. P. Matsoso, J. G. Meara, M. Mohanan, Y. Ndiaye, O. F. Norheim, K. S. Reddy, A. K. Rowe, J. A. Salomon, G. Thapa, N. A. Y. Twum-Danso, and M. Pate. 2018. High-quality health systems in the sustainable development goals era: Time for a revolution. *Lancet Global Health* 6(11):e1196–e1252.

Kupferschmidt, K. 2019. Successful Ebola treatments promise to tame outbreak. *Science* 365(6454):628–629.

Lenhart, A. 2019. *The role of innovation in the evolution of global vector control response.* PowerPoint presented at the workshop on Exploring the Frontiers of Innovation to Tackle Microbial Threats, Washington, DC.

Liu, V., M. P. Clark, M. Mendoza, R. Saket, M. N. Gardner, B. J. Turk, and G. J. Escobar. 2013. Automated identification of pneumonia in chest radiograph reports in critically ill patients. *BMC Medical Informatics and Decision Making* 13:90.

Mabud, T. S., M. de Lourdes Delgado Alves, A. I. Ko, S. Basu, K. S. Walter, T. Cohen, B. Mathema, C. Colijn, E. Lemos, J. Croda, and J. R. Andrews. 2019. Evaluating strategies for control of tuberculosis in prisons and prevention of spillover into communities: An observational and modeling study from brazil. *PLOS Medicine* 16(3).

McMullan, L. K., M. Flint, A. Chakrabarti, L. Guerrero, M. K. Lo, D. Porter, S. T. Nichol, C. F. Spiropoulou, and C. Albarino. 2019. Characterisation of infectious ebola virus from the ongoing outbreak to guide response activities in the democratic republic of the congo: A phylogenetic and in vitro analysis. *The Lancet Infectious Diseases* 19(9):1023–1032.

Meeker, D., T. K. Knight, M. W. Friedberg, J. A. Linder, N. J. Goldstein, C. R. Fox, A. Rothfeld, G. Diaz, and J. N. Doctor. 2014. Nudgying guideline-concordant antibiotic prescribing: A randomized clinical trial. *JAMA Internal Medicine* 174(3):425–431.

Moran, M., J. Guzman, K. Henderson, R. Liyanage, L. Wu, E. Chin, N. Chapman, L. Abela-Oversteegen, D. Gouglas, and D. Kwong. 2012. *Neglected disease research and development: A five year review.* Sydney, Australia: Policy Cures.

Moreira, L. A., I. Iturbe-Ormaetxe, J. A. Jeffery, G. Lu, A. T. Pyke, L. M. Hedges, B. C. Rocha, S. Hall-Mendelin, A. Day, M. Riegler, L. E. Hugo, K. N. Johnson, B. H. Kay, E. A. McGraw, A. F. van den Hurk, P. A. Ryan, and S. L. O'Neill. 2009. A *Wolbachia* symbiont in *Aedes aegypti* limits infection with dengue, chikungunya, and plasmodium. *Cell* 139(7):1268–1278.

Narra, R., J. Sobel, C. Piper, D. Gould, N. Bhadelia, M. Dott, A. Fiore, W. A. Fischer, M. J. Frawley, P. M. Griffin, D. Hamilton, B. Mahon, S. K. Pillai, E. F. Veltus, R. Tauxe, and M. Jhung. 2017. CDC safety training course for Ebola virus disease health workers. *Emerging Infectious Diseases* 23(13):S217–S224.

Ozawa, S., S. Clark, A. Portnoy, S. Grewal, M. L. Stack, A. Sinha, A. Mirelman, H. Franklin, I. K. Friberg, and Y. Tam. 2017. Estimated economic impact of vaccinations in 73 low- and middle-income countries, 2001–2020. *Bulletin of the World Health Organization* 95(9):629.

Pant Pai, N., J. Sharma, S. Shivkumar, S. Pillay, C. Vadnais, L. Joseph, K. Dheda, and R. W. Peeling. 2013a. Supervised and unsupervised self-testing for HIV in high- and low-risk populations: A systematic review. *PLOS Medicine* 10(4):e1001414.

Pant Pai, N., T. Behlim, L. Abrahams, C. Vadnais, S. Shivkumar, S. Pillay, A. Binder, R. Deli-Houssein, N. Engel, L. Joseph, and K. Dheda. 2013b. Will an unsupervised self-testing strategy for HIV work in health care workers of South Africa? A cross sectional pilot feasibility study. *PLOS ONE* 8(11):e79772.

Pant Pai, N., J. Sharma, B. Balram, M. Bhargava, S. Pillay, L. Joseph, and P. P. Tellier. 2014. Will an unsupervised self-testing strategy be feasible to operationalize in Canada? Results from a pilot study in students of a large Canadian university. *AIDS Research and Treatment* 2014:747619.

Pant Pai, N., M. Smallwood, L. Desjardins, A. Goyette, K. G. Birkas, A. F. Vassal, L. Joseph, and R. Thomas. 2018. An unsupervised smart app-optimized HIV self-testing program in Montreal, Canada: Cross-sectional study. *Journal of Medical Internet Research* 20(11):e10258.

Pettitt, J., E. Higgs, M. Fallah, M. Nason, E. Stavale, J. Marchand, C. Reilly, K. Jensen, B. Dighero-Kemp, K. Tuznik, J. Logue, F. Bolay, and L. Hensley. 2017. Assessment and optimization of the GeneXpert diagnostic platform for detection of Ebola virus RNA in seminal fluid. *Journal of Infectious Diseases* 215(4):547–553.

Platt, L. R., C. F. Estivariz, and R. W. Suttler. 2014. Vaccine-associated paralytic poliomyelitis: A review of the epidemiology and estimation of the global burden. *Journal of Infectious Diseases* 210(Suppl 1):S380–S389.

Raftery, P., O. Condell, C. Wasunna, J. Kpaka, R. Zwizwai, M. Nuha, M. Fallah, M. Freeman, V. Harris, M. Miller, A. Baller, M. Massaquoi, V. Katawera, J. Saindon, P. Bemah, E. Hamblion, E. Castle, D. Williams, A. Gasasira, T. Nyenswah, and E. Mossel. 2018. Establishing Ebola virus disease (EVD) diagnostics using genexpert technology at a mobile laboratory in Liberia: Impact on outbreak response, case management and laboratory systems strengthening. *PLOS Neglected Tropical Diseases* 12(1):e0006135.

Ribeiro, C. D. S., M. Y. van Roode, G. B. Haringhuizen, M. P. Koopmans, E. Claassen, and L. H. M. van de Burgwal. 2018a. How ownership rights over microorganisms affect infectious disease control and innovation: A root-cause analysis of barriers to data sharing as experienced by key stakeholders. *PLOS ONE* 13(5).

Ribeiro, C. D. S., M. P. Koopmans, and G. B. Haringhuizen. 2018b. Threats to timely sharing of pathogen sequence data. *Science* 362(6413):404–406.

Roberts, L. 2020. Global polio eradication falters in the final stretch. *Science* 367(6473):14–15.

Roscigno, G., Y. Yuthavong, and L. Manderson. 2012. Innovation and new technologies to tackle infectious diseases of poverty. In *Global Report for Research on Infectious Diseases of Poverty*, edited by M. Harris and J. N. Reza. Geneva, Switzerland: World Health Organization. Pp. 94–114.

Saha, S. 2019. *Unbiased metagenomic sequencing to counter microbial threats: Lessons from Bangladesh*. PowerPoint presented at the workshop on Exploring the Frontiers of Innovation to Tackle Microbial Threats, Washington, DC.

Saha, S., S. Saha, and S. K. Saha. 2018. Barriers in Bangladesh. *Elife* 7.

Saha, S., A. Ramesh, K. Kalantar, R. Malaker, M. Hasanuzzaman, L. M. Khan, M. Y. Mayday, M. S. I. Sajib, L. M. Li, C. Langelier, H. Rahman, E. D. Crawford, C. M. Tato, M. Islam, Y. F. Juan, C. de Bourcy, B. Dimitrov, J. Wang, J. Tang, J. Sheu, R. Egger, T. R. De Carvalho, M. R. Wilson, S. K. Saha, and J. L. DeRisi. 2019a. Unbiased metagenomic sequencing for pediatric meningitis in Bangladesh reveals neuroinvasive chikungunya virus outbreak and other unrealized pathogens. *mBio* 10(6).

Saha, S., M. M. H. Afrad, S. Saha, and S. K. Saha. 2019b. Towards making global health research truly global. *Lancet Global Health* 7(9):e1175.

Sands, P. 2018. *Ending epidemics and building health systems*. https://www.theglobalfund.org/en/blog/2018-10-12-ending-epidemics-and-building-health-systems (accessed March 16, 2020).

Semper, A. E., M. J. Broadhurst, J. Richards, G. M. Foster, A. J. Simpson, C. H. Logue, J. D. Kelly, A. Miller, T. J. Brooks, M. Murray, and N. R. Pollock. 2016. Performance of the GeneXpert Ebola assay for diagnosis of Ebola virus disease in Sierra Leone: A field evaluation study. *PLOS Medicine* 13(3):e1001980.

Stenberg, K., O. Hanssen, T. T. Edejer, M. Bertram, C. Brindley, A. Meshreky, J. E. Rosen, J. Stover, P. Verboom, R. Sanders, and A. Soucat. 2017. Financing transformative health systems towards achievement of the health sustainable development goals: A model for projected resource needs in 67 low-income and middle-income countries. *Lancet Global Health* 5(9):e875–e887.

Sullivan, N. J., A. Sanchez, P. E. Rollin, Z. Y. Yang, and G. J. Nabel. 2000. Development of a preventive vaccine for Ebola virus infection in primates. *Nature* 408(6812):605–609.

Swanepoel, R., S. B. Smit, P. E. Rollin, P. Formenty, P. A. Leman, A. Kemp, F. J. Burt, A. A. Grobbelaar, J. Croft, D. G. Bausch, H. Zeller, H. Leirs, L. E. Braack, M. L. Libande, S. Zaki, S. T. Nichol, T. G. Ksiazek, J. T. Paweska, S. International, and the Technical Committee for Marburg Hemorrhagic Fever Control in the Democratic Republic of the Congo. 2007. Studies of reservoir hosts for marburg virus. *Emerging Infectious Diseases* 13(12):1847–1851.

Talkington, K., C. Shore, and P. Kothari. 2016. *A scientific roadmap for antibiotic discovery.* Philiadelphia, PA: The Pew Charitable Trusts.

Thaler, R. H., and C. R. Sunstein. 2009. *Nudge: Improving decisions about health, wealth, and happiness.* New York: Penguin.

The Pew Charitable Trusts. 2018. *Achaogen provides data to SPARK, Pew's platform for antibiotic discovery research.* https://www.pewtrusts.org/en/about/news-room/press-releases-and-statements/2018/10/22/achaogen-provides-data-to-spark-pews-platform-for-antibiotic-discovery-research (accessed February 2, 2020).

The Pew Charitable Trusts. 2019a. *Tracking the global pipeline of antibiotics in development.* https://www.pewtrusts.org/en/research-and-analysis/issue-briefs/2019/09/tracking-the-global-pipeline-of-antibiotics-in-development (accessed March 5, 2020).

The Pew Charitable Trusts. 2019b. *Novartis provides data to SPARK, Pew's platform for antibiotic discovery research.* https://www.pewtrusts.org/en/about/news-room/press-releases-and-statements/2019/01/03/novartis-provides-data-to-spark-pews-platform-for-antibiotic-discovery-research (accessed February 2, 2020).

The Pew Charitable Trusts. 2019c. *Novartis shares 2 new datasets with SPARK, Pew's antibiotic discovery tool.* https://www.pewtrusts.org/en/research-and-analysis/articles/2019/05/10/novartis-shares-2-new-datasets-with-spark-pews-antibiotic-discovery-tool (accessed February 2, 2020).

Towner, J. S. 2019. *Advancing innovation on the ground in the fight against Ebola (a CDC perspective).* PowerPoint presented at the workshop on Exploring the Frontiers of Innovation to Tackle Microbial Threats, Washington, DC.

Towner, J. S., T. K. Sealy, M. L. Khristova, C. G. Albarino, S. Conlan, S. A. Reeder, P. L. Quan, W. I. Lipkin, R. Downing, J. W. Tappero, S. Okware, J. Lutwama, B. Bakamutumaho, J. Kayiwa, J. A. Comer, P. E. Rollin, T. G. Ksiazek, and S. T. Nichol. 2008. Newly discovered Ebola virus associated with hemorrhagic fever outbreak in Uganda. *PLOS Pathogens* 4(11):e1000212.

Towner, J. S., B. R. Amman, T. K. Sealy, S. A. Carroll, J. A. Comer, A. Kemp, R. Swanepoel, C. D. Paddock, S. Balinandi, M. L. Khristova, P. B. Formenty, C. G. Albarino, D. M. Miller, Z. D. Reed, J. T. Kayiwa, J. N. Mills, D. L. Cannon, P. W. Greer, E. Byaruhanga, E. C. Farnon, P. Atimnedi, S. Okware, E. Katongole-Mbidde, R. Downing, J. W. Tappero, S. R. Zaki, T. G. Ksiazek, S. T. Nichol, and P. E. Rollin. 2009. Isolation of genetically diverse Marburg viruses from Egyptian fruit bats. *PLOS Pathogens* 5(7):e1000536.

UNAIDS (Joint United Nations Programme on HIV/AIDS). 2014. *90-90-90: An ambitious treatment target to help end the AIDS epidemic.* Geneva, Switzerland: Joint United Nations Programme on HIV/AIDS.

USAID (U.S. Agency for International Development). 2019a. *Private-sector engagement evidence and learning plan.* https://www.usaid.gov/work-usaid/private-sector-engagement/evidence-and-learning-plan (accessed February 2, 2020).

USAID. 2019b. *Private-sector engagement policy.* https://www.usaid.gov/sites/default/files/documents/1865/usaid_psepolicy_final.pdf (accessed February 2, 2020).

Van Damme, P., I. Coster, A. S. Bandyopadhyay, L. Suykens, P. Rudelsheim, P. Neels, M. S. Oberste, W. C. Weldon, R. Clemens, and H. Revets. 2019a. Poliopolis: Pushing boundaries of scientific innovations for disease eradication. *Future Microbiology* 14(15):1321–1330.

Van Damme, P., I. De Coster, A. S. Bandyopadhyay, H. Revets, K. Withanage, P. De Smedt, L. Suykens, M. S. Oberste, W. C. Weldon, S. A. Costa-Clemens, R. Clemens, J. Modlin, A. J. Weiner, A. J. Macadam, R. Andino, O. M. Kew, J. L. Konopka-Anstadt, C. C. Burns, J. Konz, R. Wahid, and C. Gast. 2019b. The safety and immunogenicity of two novel live attenuated monovalent (serotype 2) oral poliovirus vaccines in healthy adults: A double-blind, single-centre phase 1 study. *Lancet* 394(10193):148–158.

van den Hurk, A. F., S. Hall-Mendelin, A. T. Pyke, F. D. Frentiu, K. McElroy, A. Day, S. Higgs, and S. L. O'Neill. 2012. Impact of *Wolbachia* on infection with chikungunya and yellow fever viruses in the mosquito vector *Aedes aegypti. PLOS Neglected Tropical Diseases* 6(11):e1892.

van Vuren, P. J., A. Grobbelaar, N. Storm, O. Conteh, K. Konneh, A. Kamara, I. Sanne, and J. T. Paweska. 2016. Comparative evaluation of the diagnostic performance of the prototype Cepheid GeneXpert Ebola assay. *Journal of Clinical Microbiology* 54(2):359–367.

Wesolowski, A., T. Qureshi, M. F. Boni, P. R. Sundsoy, M. A. Johansson, S. B. Rasheed, K. Engo-Monsen, and C. O. Buckee. 2015. Impact of human mobility on the emergence of dengue epidemics in Pakistan. *Proceedings of the National Academy of Sciences of the United States of America* 112(38):11887–11892.

WHO (World Health Organization). 2015. *Global action plan on antimicrobial resistance.* https://apps.who.int/iris/handle/10665/193736 (accessed March 5, 2020).

WHO. 2016. *HIV self-testing and partner notification.* Geneva, Switzerland: World Health Organization.

WHO. 2017a. *Global vector control response 2017–2030.* Geneva, Switzerland: World Health Organization.

WHO. 2017b. *Invasive bacterial vaccine preventable diseases laboratory network.* https://www.who.int/immunization/monitoring_surveillance/burden/laboratory/IBVPD/en (accessed March 3, 2020).

WHO. 2018a. *World malaria report 2018.* Geneva, Switzerland: World Health Organization.

WHO. 2018b. *Resource mobilisation for antimicrobial resistance (AMR): Getting AMR into plans and budgets of government and development partners: Nepal country report.* Geneva, Switzerland: World Health Organization.

WHO. 2019a. *Poliomyelitis: Key facts.* https://www.who.int/news-room/fact-sheets/detail/poliomyelitis (accessed February 20, 2020).

WHO. 2019b. *Two out of three wild poliovirus strains eradicated.* https://www.who.int/news-room/feature-stories/detail/two-out-of-three-wild-poliovirus-strains-eradicated (accessed February 20, 2020).

WHO. 2019c. *What is vaccine-derived polio?* https://www.who.int/features/qa/64/en (accessed February 20, 2020).

WHO. 2019d. *HIV self-testing.* https://www.who.int/hiv/topics/self-testing/en (accessed March 4, 2020).

WHO. 2019e. *WHO guidelines on tuberculosis infection prevention and control.* Geneva, Switzerland: World Health Organization.

WHO. 2019f. *Immunization coverage: Key facts.* https://www.who.int/news-room/fact-sheets/detail/immunization-coverage (accessed February 20, 2020).

WHO. 2019g. *Turning plans into action for antimicrobial resistance (AMR)—Working paper 2.0: Implementation and coordination.* Geneva, Switzerland: World Health Organization.

WHO. 2020. *Ebola virus disease: Key facts.* https://www.who.int/news-room/fact-sheets/detail/ebola-virus-disease (accessed March 3, 2020).

Ye, Y. H., A. M. Carrasco, F. D. Frentiu, S. F. Chenoweth, N. W. Beebe, A. F. van den Hurk, C. P. Simmons, S. L. O'Neill, and E. A. McGraw. 2015. *Wolbachia* reduces the transmission potential of dengue-infected *Aedes aegypti. PLOS Neglected Tropical Diseases* 9(6):e0003894.

Yozwiak, N. L., S. F. Schaffner, and P. C. Sabeti. 2015. Data sharing: Make outbreak research open access. *Nature* 518(7540):477–479.

Appendix A

Workshop Statement of Task

This is a 1.5-day public workshop designed to examine the major advancements in scientific, technological, and social innovations that have been taking place to tackle microbial threats, including diagnostics, vaccine development and production, and new antimicrobials as well as nonpharmaceutical interventions and surveillance. The workshop will offer particular consideration to innovations that occur at the human–animal–plant–environment interface and those that are practical and can be implemented in different resource-level settings.

Specifically, this workshop will feature invited presentations and discussions including the following:

- Detection and diagnostic tools that empower end users and patients to take appropriate action including obtaining early treatment;
- Cutting-edge methods and tools such as advances in predictive modeling, digital platforms, and precision public health, and how to best make use of them in practice;
- Novel innovations that take into account social and behavioral factors related to microbial threats;
- Communication and structural strategies that would help demystify the uptake and increase access of effective innovations to facilitate positive behavior change and strengthen preparedness and response capacities;
- Approaches to leverage data and modeling insights that would be useful for practitioners working on the ground in diverse settings, particularly at the community level;

- Models and indicators that help reveal the extent to which the innovations are "successful"; and
- Effective mechanisms for stimulating meaningful collaboration and communication among various stakeholders, including multilateral organizations, national governments, private sector, and civil society.

Workshop speakers and discussants will contribute perspectives from government, academia, private, and nonprofit sectors.

Appendix B

Workshop Agenda

Exploring the Frontiers of Innovation to Tackle Microbial Threats: A Workshop

December 4–5, 2019

Keck Center
500 Fifth Street, NW
Washington, DC 20001

DAY 1—WEDNESDAY, DECEMBER 4, 2019

1:00 pm ET Welcome Remarks
Peter Daszak, EcoHealth Alliance

Workshop Overview and Goals
Kent Kester, Sanofi Pasteur
Rafael Obregón, United Nations Children's Fund

Keynote Addresses
Applying Lessons Learned from Innovation in Polio Eradication
Ananda Bandyopadhyay, Bill & Melinda Gates Foundation

Advancing Innovation on the Ground in the Fight Against Ebola
Jonathan Towner, U.S. Centers for Disease Control and Prevention

Q&A

Session I: Harnessing Lessons from Emerging Scientific, Technological, and Social Innovations

Greg Armstrong, U.S. Centers for Disease Control and Prevention, *Moderator*

2:00 pm	The Role of Innovation in the Evolution of Global Vector Control Response **Audrey Lenhart,** U.S. Centers for Disease Control and Prevention
	Applying Modeling to Inform Infectious Disease Surveillance and Outbreak Response **Caroline Buckee,** Center for Communicable Disease Dynamics, Harvard T.H. Chan School of Public Health
	Unbiased Metagenomics Sequencing to Counter Microbial Threats: Lessons from Bangladesh **Senjuti Saha,** Child Health Research Foundation
	Will Process Innovations for HIV Self-Testing Impact Health Outcomes at the Community Level? **Nitika Pant Pai,** McGill University
3:00 pm	Q&A
3:30 pm	Break

Session II: Overcoming Barriers in the Field to Bolster Access and Practical Use of Innovations

Eva Harris, University of California, Berkeley, *Moderator*

3:45 pm	Empowering Health Workers to Improve Immunization Service Delivery Through Digital Innovation **Collince Osewe,** ChanjoPlus

	Translating Data and Modeling Insights into Improved Capacity for Detection and Response **Brian Bird,** University of California, Davis
	Fostering Collaboration and Practical Tools to Enhance Timely Sharing of Data **Carolina Dos S. Ribeiro,** Centre for Infectious Disease Control, The Netherlands
	Applying Insights from Behavioral Sciences to Enhance Acceptability and Adoption of Innovations Across Diverse Social and Cultural Contexts **Fadi Makki,** Nudge Lebanon and Consumer Citizen Lab
4:45 pm	Q&A
5:15 pm	Observations from Day 1 **Kent Kester,** Sanofi Pasteur
5:30 pm	Adjourn

DAY 2—THURSDAY, DECEMBER 5, 2019

8:15 am ET	Welcome and Recap of Day 1 **Rafael Obregón,** United Nations Children's Fund

Session III: Taking a Systems Approach to Spur Innovation in Tackling Antimicrobial Resistance

	Cristina Cassetti, National Institute of Allergy and Infectious Diseases, *Moderator*
8:25 am	Lessons from One Health: Enhancing Animal and Human Surveillance Systems to Bolster Innovation in Antimicrobial Resistance **Christine Kreuder Johnson,** University of California, Davis
	Sparking Antibiotic Discover Through Data Sharing and Scientific Collaboration **Wes Kim,** The Pew Charitable Trusts

Incentivizing Novel Diagnostic Tests to Counter Antibiotic Resistance
Daniel Berman, Longitude Prize

Strengthening Health Systems to Overcome Market and Regulatory Barriers to Innovation on Antimicrobial Resistance
Jyoti Joshi, Center for Disease Dynamics, Economics & Policy

9:20 am Q&A

9:50 am Break

Session IV: Translating Innovation into Convergent Action

Part A: Overcoming Barriers and Forging Partnerships

Alan Tennenberg, Johnson & Johnson Global Public Health, *Moderator*

10:05 am **Matthew Hepburn,** U.S. Army
Rahima Dosani, U.S. Agency for International Development
Rajeev Venkayya, Global Vaccine Unit, Takeda Pharmaceuticals

11:15 am Q&A

12:00 pm Lunch

Part B: Incubating Action Through Novel Ecosystems

Rick Bright, Biomedical Advanced Research and Development Authority, *Moderator*

1:00 pm **Sabrina Welsh,** Human Vaccines Project
Maurizio Vecchione, Intellectual Ventures
Sally Allain, JLABS
Ranga Sampath, Foundation for Innovative New Diagnostics

2:00 pm Q&A

2:45 pm Break

Visionary Statements on Priorities for Innovation

Marcos Espinal, Pan American Health Organization, *Moderator*

3:00 pm **Julio Croda,** Secretary of Health Surveillance, Brazil
Carrie Teicher, Doctors Without Borders/Médecins Sans Frontières
Lori Burrows, Michael G. DeGroote Institute for Infectious Disease Research
Peter Sands, The Global Fund to Fight AIDS, Tuberculosis and Malaria

3:30 pm Final Synthesis and Discussion with Audience

4:10 pm Closing Remarks
Kent Kester, Sanofi Pasteur
Peter Daszak, EcoHealth Alliance

4:30 pm Adjourn

Appendix C

Speaker Biographies

Sally Allain, M.Sc., M.B.A., is the Head of JLABS @ Washington, DC. Ms. Allain sets the strategic direction and oversees all operational activities for JLABS in the greater Washington metro region, including Maryland and Virginia. In addition to managing the business of JLABS, Ms. Allain is responsible for the process of evaluating, selecting, and accelerating a strong portfolio of innovators for JLABS @ Washington, DC. Drawing on 18 years of experience, Ms. Allain is creating strategic partnerships with corporate, academic, government, and industry organizations, building a strong and dynamic network of innovation for patients and consumers. Ms. Allain joined JLABS after serving as Senior Director, Strategy & Operations, on the Global External Innovation team at Johnson & Johnson, where she drove global external portfolio management and reporting while leading cross-sector engagement, as well as supporting strategic business plan development. Prior, Ms. Allain built a research operations and alliance management team within Immunology to support an early discovery research and development portfolio. She also has experience in roles driving strategic initiatives in translational medicine, the development of partnerships with the Johnson & Johnson Innovation Centers, and driving teams to enhance a positive corporate culture. In addition to her career at Johnson & Johnson, Ms. Allain has had experience in biotech start-ups, as well as working internationally with ITI Life Sciences, a UK governmental economic development agency aimed at developing innovative early-stage biotech and academic collaborative programs. Ms. Allain received her M.B.A. from the University of California, Berkeley, Haas School of Business; an M.Sc. in microbiology/immunology from Virginia Tech; and a B.S. in biology from Virginia Tech.

Ananda Bandyopadhyay, M.B.B.S., M.P.H., considers himself a foot soldier in the battle to eradicate diseases. Dr. Bandyopadhyay grew up in Kolkata, India, and completed his medical graduation from Calcutta National Medical College & Hospital (2005). He received his M.P.H. in global health from the Harvard T.H. Chan School of Public Health (2010). In between (2006–2009), he worked for the polio eradication initiative in India as a Surveillance Medical Officer with the National Polio Surveillance Project of the World Health Organization, and contributed to India's successful and historic polio elimination effort and measles surveillance initiatives. He worked as an Infectious Disease Epidemiologist at Rhode Island State Department of Health in the United States for 2 years before joining the Bill & Melinda Gates Foundation in 2012. As a Senior Program Officer at the Gates Foundation, he supports global polio vaccine research and product development initiatives across multiple countries and geographies. His research is focused on generating data regarding the best use of polio vaccines to make them affordable and accessible to vulnerable and underserved populations. He is also involved in enhancing and expanding polio environmental surveillance globally with newer tools and diagnostics. His work on clinical development of novel polio vaccines and on polio endgame vaccination schedules has been a factor in global policy formulation and has been published in leading peer-reviewed journals. He is associated with advanced degree programs in public health and vaccinology in several globally renowned teaching venues as a guest faculty member.

Daniel Berman heads up the Global Health team at Nesta Challenges, including managing the Longitude Prize, which is a £10 million project designed to incentivize the development of a rapid diagnostic test to improve the use of antibiotics internationally. Mr. Berman represents Nesta in international One Health forums designed to address the challenge of antimicrobial resistance (AMR). This includes championing new strategies to address the market failure that has led to a lack of diagnostic products to address AMR. He is also exploring new prizes in essential surgery and nonpharmaceutical treatments of chronic pain. Before coming to Nesta, Mr. Berman was a consultant for the World Health Organization in Ethiopia on a local pharmaceutical production project. Previously he was at Médecins Sans Frontières (MSF) for more than 16 years. At MSF he had multiple assignments in the Access to Medicines Campaign, which focuses on stimulating and steering innovation and access to medicines, diagnostics, and vaccines. From 2012 to 2015 Mr. Berman was the General Director of MSF Southern Africa, based in Johannesburg, South Africa. He is currently a Trustee for QUAMED, a French nongovernmental organization that supports humanitarian organizations and national procurement institutions to improve the quality of medicines.

Brian Bird, D.V.M., M.P.H., Ph.D., leads Ebola-related surveillance activities as part of the U.S. Agency for International Development–funded PREDICT program led by the University of California, Davis (UC Davis). Dr. Bird's work has a particular focus in Guinea, Liberia, and Sierra Leone to identify the animal reservoir origins of ebolaviruses, and to determine if spillover into other animal species occurred during the recent devastating regional outbreak. He is Co-principal Investigator for the Defense Advanced Research Project Agency–funded Preventing Emerging Pandemic Threats project at UC Davis, where he leads in-depth investigations of Lassa fever virus ecology, genomics, and spillover dynamics from rodent reservoirs into humans in West Africa. Previously, Dr. Bird served as a veterinary medical officer for the U.S. Centers for Disease Control and Prevention (CDC) Viral Special Pathogens Branch. He was an early-stage lead of the CDC Emergency Operations Center Laboratory task force during the 2014–2016 West African Ebola epidemic, and then later lead of the CDC field-diagnostic laboratory in Sierra Leone, which successfully and safely tested more than 27,000 specimens from suspected Ebola virus patients

Caroline Buckee M.Res., D.Phil., is an Associate Professor of epidemiology and the Associate Director of the Center for Communicable Disease Dynamics at the Harvard T.H. Chan School of Public Health. She has been working to understand and control infectious diseases among the world's most vulnerable populations—in particular malaria—since obtaining her D.Phil. from Merton College, Oxford University, in 2006. Following her graduate training, Dr. Buckee won a Sir Henry Wellcome Postdoctoral Fellowship to study malaria in Kenya, and an Omidyar Fellowship at the Santa Fe Institute to harness complex systems approaches in her research. Dr. Buckee's group is interested in how the ecological and evolutionary aspects of infectious disease transmission lead to patterns of disease in human populations, particularly how human mobility affects the spread of infection. Her group pioneered the use of mobile phone "big data" and pathogen genomics to measure population movement patterns that drive epidemics. She works with malaria control programs and ministries of health in Bangladesh, Colombia, Guyana, India, and Thailand to translate these new data-driven approaches into surveillance and forecasting tools. Most recently, Dr. Buckee led a team to estimate the impact of Hurricane Maria on mortality in Puerto Rico, which was the most widely cited article of 2018. Her work has appeared in high-profile scientific journals such as *Science*, *Nature*, and the *Proceedings of the National Academy of Sciences of the United States of America*, and in the popular press, including CNN, *The New Scientist*, NPR, BBC, Radio 4, and Voice of America. She was chosen as one of *MIT Technology Review*'s 35 Innovators Under 35, a CNN Top 10: Thinker, and one of *Foreign Policy Magazine*'s Global Thinkers.

Lori Burrows, Ph.D., is a microbiologist and international authority on the structure, function, and regulation of type IV pili (T4P), ubiquitous bacterial virulence factors used for adherence, DNA uptake, biofilm formation, and twitching motility. Using the opportunistic pathogen *Pseudomonas aeruginosa* as a model, her group studies its pilin repertoire (relevant to vaccine design), pilin glycosylation systems involved in bacteriophage defense, structure–function of the pilus assembly system and its integration into the cell envelope, and the complex regulation underlying T4P function. Her lab also studies biofilm formation, particularly stimulation of biofilm development by subinhibitory antibiotic concentrations and exploitation of the stimulation phenotype to find new antimicrobials for multidrug-resistant gram-negative bacteria. Dr. Burrows's research is funded by the Canadian Institutes of Health Research (CIHR), the Natural Sciences and Engineering Research Council of Canada, the Canadian Glycomics Network, the Ontario Research Fund, and industrial support. She has published more than 100 peer-reviewed papers, reviews, and book chapters. She is the Associate Director (Partnerships and Outreach) of McMaster's Michael G. DeGroote Institute for Infectious Disease Research and serves on the editorial boards of the *Journal of Bacteriology*, the *Journal of Biochemistry*, and the American Chemical Society's *Infectious Diseases*. She served as Chair (2010–2017) of the CIHR Microbiology and Infectious Diseases Peer-Review Panel, the Scientific Officer of Cystic Fibrosis Canada's biomedical grants panel, a member of the Polyani Prize panel, and McMaster University's CIHR University Delegate since 2012. In 2017 she was elected as a Fellow of the American Academy of Microbiology.

Julio Croda, M.D., Ph.D., is the Chief of the Department of Communicable Diseases at the Secretary of Health Surveillance in Brazil. He is an infectious disease physician-scientist and has served as the Principal Investigator for a series of studies involving active surveillance, molecular epidemiology, and prospective cohort investigations for tuberculosis (TB). He is particularly interested in understanding how prisons contribute globally to TB epidemics, with an ultimate goal of developing more effective interventions to control TB in prisons and communities using translational research and implementation science. Dr. Croda's training is in epidemiology and clinical medicine, and his work includes epidemiology, fieldwork, and analysis of programmatic data. His research program is currently funded by the National Institutes of Health and by Brazilian research agencies such as the National Council for Scientific and Technological Development and Coordenação de Aperfeiçoamento de Pessoal de Nível Superior.

Rahima Dosani, M.P.H., M.B.A., is a market access advisor at the Center for Innovation and Impact with the U.S. Agency for International Development's (USAID's) Bureau for Global Health. She works on increasing access to global health commodities while improving the functioning of global health markets across disease areas through market shaping efforts, innovative financing structures, private-sector engagement, supply chain improvement, digital health interventions, and human-centered design efforts. Prior to USAID, Ms. Dosani worked at FSG, a social impact consulting firm, where she led global health, international development, and corporate consulting projects. She spent several years living in Malawi and Myanmar working for the Clinton Health Access Initiative, where she served as a technical and strategic advisor to the Ministry of Health to accelerate the introduction of new vaccines, HIV diagnostics, and tuberculosis treatment into both countries. Ms. Dosani began her career in the public sector and health care consulting at PricewaterhouseCoopers Advisory in New York City. She graduated summa cum laude from the University of Pennsylvania, where she studied global health and health care management. Ms. Dosani also holds an M.B.A. from the Harvard Business School and an M.P.H. in global health from the Harvard T.H. Chan School of Public Health, where she was a Zuckerman Fellow through the Harvard University Center for Public Leadership. Ms. Dosani is passionate about social justice, gender equity, and spreading empathy, compassion, and vulnerability to make the world a better place.

Matthew Hepburn, M.D., is the joint product lead at the U.S. Army. He joined the Defense Advanced Research Projects Agency (DARPA) as a Program Manager in 2013. He aims to address the dynamic threats of emerging infectious diseases with potential impact on national security. Prior to joining DARPA, COL Hepburn served as the Director of Medical Preparedness on the White House National Security Staff. Additional previous assignments include Chief Medical Officer at a Level II medical facility in Iraq, Clinical Research Director at the U.S. Army Medical Research Institute for Infectious Diseases, Exchange Officer to the United Kingdom, and Internal Medicine Chief of Residents at Brooke Army Medical Center at Fort Sam Houston, Texas. COL Hepburn completed internal medicine residency and infectious diseases fellowship programs at Brooke Army Medical Center. He holds an M.D. and a B.S. in biomedical engineering from Duke University.

Christine Kreuder Johnson, V.M.D., M.P.V.M., Ph.D., is a professor of epidemiology at the University of California, Davis, and is dedicated to advancing disease investigations at the interface of animal, human, and environmental health through applied research to inform disease prevention and pandemic preparedness. Research activities have sought to investigate the dynamics of high-priority zoonoses and understand the human dimensions of spillover, providing insight for policy changes needed to mitigate risk and prevent epidemics. She is the Co-principal Investigator of the U.S. Agency for International Development's (USAID's) Emerging Pandemic Threats PREDICT program, a 10-year project to detect emerging threats and enhance pandemic preparedness in more than 30 countries, for which she directs surveillance activities in humans and animals. As a multi-institutional consortium, PREDICT has partnered with host country governments to establish an international network of scientists engaged in pathogen discovery, risk characterization, and outbreak response. She has pioneered ecosystem-level studies to investigate the impact of environmental change on population health, and contributes expertise to outbreak investigations at the request of state, federal, and international agencies, including USAID, the U.S. Department of Defense, the California Department of Fish and Wildlife, and the U.S. Fish & Wildlife Service.

Jyoti Joshi, M.D., M.Sc., is the Head of the South Asia Center for Disease Dynamics, Economics & Policy. She has an M.D. with a specialization in community medicine and an M.Sc. in infectious diseases from the London School of Hygiene & Tropical Medicine, University of London. She is also an Adjunct Professor at the Amity Institute of Public Health, Amity University, Noida, India. Dr. Joshi leads several academic research projects in the field of antimicrobial resistance, maternal and child health, immunization, and vaccine safety. As the South Asia lead for the Global Antibiotic Research Partnership (GARP) project, she has supported GARP country working groups to develop antimicrobial resistance (AMR) situation analyses and national action plans. She has advised the World Health Organization in developing guidance for implementing national action plans for AMR. Dr. Joshi co-authored the *Scoping Report* on the AMR research landscape in India, and is currently implementing two Department of Biotechnology–funded AMR projects in India: "Smart Regulation of Antibiotics in India—Understanding, Innovating, and Improving Compliance," and "Chicken or Egg: Drivers of Antimicrobial Resistance in Poultry in India (DARPI)." During the course of more than a decade and a half, Dr. Joshi has helped strengthen disease surveillance, immunization, and vaccine pharmacovigilance programs in India and the United Arab Emirates.

Wes Kim, Ph.D., M.B.A., leads efforts to spur the innovation of new antibiotics for Pew's antibiotic resistance project. His work focuses on research and policies that will help to advance antibiotic discovery and development. Before joining Pew, Dr. Kim was a management consultant in the pharmaceutical and life sciences industry, advising clients on research and development strategy and operations, with a focus on infectious diseases. His clients included multinational companies, philanthropic and donor organizations, U.S. government agencies, and nongovernmental organizations. Before that, he was a scientist at a biotech start-up, where he led development of a diagnostic kit for breast cancer. Dr. Kim has a bachelor's degree in biochemistry and religion from Oberlin College and an M.B.A. and a Ph.D. in pharmaceutical sciences from the University of Maryland.

Audrey Lenhart, Ph.D., M.P.H., is a research entomologist at the U.S. Centers for Disease Control and Prevention (CDC) in Atlanta, Georgia. She is based in the Entomology Branch of the Division of Parasitic Diseases and Malaria in the Center for Global Health, where she leads the Insecticide Resistance and Vector Control Team. Dr. Lenhart coordinates the entomology activities in the U.S. Agency for International Development–funded Latin America and Caribbean Regional Malaria Program and managed CDC's portfolio of international vector-related activities for Zika. Her team provides technical assistance throughout the Americas, Asia, and Africa regarding vector surveillance and control. She leads a research group that focuses on the biology and control of mosquitoes, and her laboratory activities aim to identify the molecular mechanisms that cause insecticide resistance in mosquito vectors of human disease. Dr. Lenhart is a founding member of the Pan American Health Organization's Technical Advisory Group for Public Health Entomology in the Americas, and is a member of the World Health Organization's Vector Control Advisory Group. She is an Honorary Research Fellow at the Liverpool School of Tropical Medicine and adjunct faculty in the Department of Environmental Sciences at Emory University.

Fadi Makki, Ph.D., is the Founder of Nudge Lebanon and the Consumer Citizen Lab. He is a pioneer in the application of behavioral economics to public policy in the Middle East and heads the first nudge unit in the Middle East, B4Development (formerly the Qatar Behavioral Insights Unit). He led a large number of randomized controlled trials and behavioral experiments across the Middle East in a variety of policy areas, including health, education, social cohesion, and inclusion. He served between 2016 and 2018 as a member of the World Economic Forum's Council for the Future of Behavioral Sciences, and is currently a Senior Fellow at Georgetown Qatar and the American University of Beirut's (AUB's) Issam Fares Institute of Public Policy. He was Director General of the Lebanese Ministry of Economy & Trade, adviser to the Lebanese Prime Minister. He was previously adviser to the Ministry of Economy and Commerce in Qatar. He worked previously at Booz & Co., and was a visiting fellow/lecturer at the Graduate Institute for International Studies in Geneva, the Lauterpacht Centre at Cambridge University, AUB, and Université Saint Joseph. He earned his Ph.D. from Cambridge University, his master's from the London School of Economics and Hull University, his bachelor's degrees from AUB, and his LLB from the Lebanese University. B4Development is the first behavioral insights and nudge unit in the Middle East, created by the Supreme Committee for Delivery and Legacy, and focusing on policy experimentation, capacity building, and the promotion of the use of evidence-based policy making, such as through behavioral sciences tools and research methods. Nudge Lebanon is a nongovernmental and nonprofit initiative working to apply behavioral insights to the policy challenges that Lebanon faces, using rigorous experimental approaches and tools typically used in the field of behavioral economics, such as randomized controlled trials. Nudge Lebanon is a leader in applying behavioral science to a variety of public policy settings, in particular, improving citizen-centered policies and steering people and organizations toward making the most optimal choices for themselves and their communities.

Collince Osewe is a budding social entrepreneur with both business and software engineering backgrounds. He believes that technology can play a critical role in bridging the inequality gap in child health, especially in enabling last mile access to lifesaving vaccines for the poor, most vulnerable, and highly mobile and impermanent communities. He holds a B.Com. (marketing) degree from the University of Nairobi. He is also well versed in social entrepreneurship, with key competencies in financial modeling for the social sector, marketing to the bottom of the pyramid, measuring social impact, as well as business models for social impact. Having worked at leading social enterprises in Kenya, he has a wealth of experience in project management, including user-centered design approaches, which has been at the core of the ChanjoPlus model. As the Founder and Chief Executive Officer at ChanjoPlus, Mr. Osewe leads strategic planning, partnership development, and fundraising strategy at ChanjoPlus. His motivation to transform the lives of children emanates from a personal experience he had during one of the immunization drives in Nairobi, Kenya, where the majority of children in high mobile urban centers missed their vaccinations and subsequently discontinued their routine immunization schedules due to lack of proper identification, making it a nightmare for health care workers to track which children were falling through the immunization gaps. He created ChanjoPlus to solve this challenge and ensure that every child has access to lifesaving vaccines no matter where they live. Through the ChanjoPlus platform, every registered child is assigned a digital identity that allows health care workers to track which children are missing out on their routine immunization services in real time.

Nitika Pant Pai, M.D., M.P.H., Ph.D., is a tenured Associate Professor at McGill University's Department of Medicine, Division of Clinical Epidemiology, and Physician Scientist at the Research Institute of the McGill University Health Centre. She is also a member of the New College of Arts

& Sciences of the Royal Society of Canada. Her Global Implementation Research program in Canada, India, and South Africa is focused on point-of-care diagnostics for HIV and associated co-infections (hepatitis C virus [HCV], hepatitis B virus [HBV], human papillomavirus [HPV], and bacterial sexually transmitted infections). Her research informs domestic and global policy on point-of-care diagnostics. She develops and incorporates innovation, implementation science, and artificial intelligence to generate solutions that plug health service delivery gaps. She strives to generate clinical, public health, and social impact. Her innovations are being implemented nationally and internationally. She has been a recipient of many research and innovation awards: Canadian Institutes of Health Research (CIHR) New Investigator award 2010, Fonds de la recherche en santé du Québec (FRSQ) Chercheur Boursier awards 2015, FRSQ senior, 2018, Grand Challenges Canada's (GCC's) Stars in Global Health Awards (2011, 2013, 2016), GCC's Transition to Scale Award (2015), McMaster University's Chanchalani Award for Research Excellence in HIV 2012, and McGill University's Maude Abbott Award for Research Excellence 2013, among others. Her research has been supported by grants from the CIHR, the FRSQ Quebec, Grand Challenges Canada, Bill & Melinda Gates Foundation, South African Medical Research Council Strategic Health Innovation Partnerships, and South African Department of Science and Technology. In 2015, she founded a social enterprise, Sympact-X, to take her innovations to scale nationally and internationally. She serves on many technical working groups for national and international agencies: the World Health Organization (WHO), Foundation for Innovative Diagnostics, Geneva; Population Services International Washington; Gates Foundation, Seattle; African Society for Laboratory Medicine (ASLM), Africa; the U.S. Centers for Disease Control and Prevention (CDC)/President's Emergency Plan for AIDS Relief (PEPFAR), Atlanta; Public Health Agency of Canada, Health Canada, and CIHR REACH. She has advised the U.S. Congress on multiplex testing for sexually transmitted and blood-borne infection (STBBI). In terms of global policies, she has also contributed to ASLM/CDC/PEPFAR's policies on quality of point-of-care testing (POCT), WHO's global HIV self-testing guidelines, and WHO's policy guidance on implementation of HIV self-testing and U.S. policies for POCTs for HIV/STBBI. She has led many systematic reviews to inform the gaps in policies for POCT and on innovations for the Joint United Nations Programme on HIV/AIDS 90-90-90 initiative to end the HIV epidemic. In Canada, she has contributed to the CIHR-REACH–funded national action plan for HIV/STBBI testing. She is a past Co-Chair of the CIHR Reach POCT 2.0 national working group and is working collaboratively to help improve the uptake of POCTs in Canada. As part of these collaborations, she is leading/co-leading three projects: approval of an HIV INSTI self-test; HIVSmart!, a Canada-wide scale up; and AideSmart!, an app-based screening of multiple co-infections (HCV, syphilis, and HBV) across key Canadian provinces. Funded by Grand Challenges Canada, she and her team developed the world's first app-based solution for HIV self-testing—the HIVSmart! app—a portable, multilingual, global screening application and platform, which won the ASAP Innovation award ($30,000) from Google, *PLOS*, and Wellcome Trust at the World Bank in 2013. She has evaluated the HIVSmart! strategy in South Africa/Canada successfully in 3,000 different at risk populations in large-scale implementation studies. The strategy is being adopted by the International Association of Providers of AIDS Care to take to scale in many fast track cities. HIVSmart! has been recently funded to be scaled across Canada. Another app-based strategy to increase the uptake of point-of-care testing by health care workers called AideSmart! (funded by Grand Challenges Canada) has proven results from India. It has been recently funded by CIHR for implementation in Canadian provinces. Funded by the India-Canada Centre for Innovative Multidisciplinary Partnerships to Accelerate Community Transformation and Sustainability, this strategy is being scaled up in at-risk populations in South India. Another of her app-based solutions, HCVSmart!, is a rapid and self-screening strategy for HCV and was featured in the Changemakers section of *The Economist* in 2017. Her work has been featured in the national and international media: *The Economist*, *MacLeans*, *The Globe and Mail*, *Montreal Gazette*, *Times Now*, *Times*, CTV, CBC, La Presse, and Radio Canada, among others.

Carolina dos S. Ribeiro, M.Sc., Ph.D. candidate, studied veterinary medicine (at the Federal University of Goiás, Brazil) and global health (at the Vrije Universiteit [VU University] Amsterdam, the Netherlands). She works as a policy advisor at the Dutch National Centre for Infectious Disease Control at the Netherlands National Institute for Public Health and the Environment, and is an external Ph.D. student leasing with the Athena Institute from the School of Earth and Life Sciences at the VU University, Amsterdam. Ms. Ribeiro participated as a junior scientist in the COMPARE project, where she researched and produced three reports on addressing the PEARL (political, ethical, administrative, regulatory, and legal) barriers to the sharing of microbial and pathogen genetic data. This involves inter alia in-depth study on ownership barriers to the sharing of microbial genetic resources, performance of workshops with different organizations on the topic of global data sharing, research on the impact of the Nagoya Protocol on the sharing of genetic resources through biobanks and culture collections, research on barriers to the design and implementation of One Health initiatives, and finally research on innovation and product valorization in the field of infectious disease response and control. Currently, Ms. Ribeiro is working on two European and international projects of EVAg (European

Virus Archive goes Global) and VEO (Versatile Emerging infectious disease Observatory). In these projects she is performing research on the implementation of the Nagoya Protocol in a global decentralized collection of microorganisms addressing ethical, legal, and administrative challenges; and on the ethical, legal, and social implications of combining big data with traditional epidemiological and molecular data for enhancing infectious disease management, including through the performance of citizen-aided science.

Senjuti Saha, Ph.D., is a Bangladeshi-Canadian microbiologist working at the intersection of clinical microbiology and global health as a scientist at the Child Health Research Foundation in Bangladesh. After completing her Ph.D. in molecular genetics at the University of Toronto in Canada, she moved back to Bangladesh to pursue a career that brings together basic science and public health. Dr. Saha's work is grounded in advancing the cause of health and research equity—she believes that everyone across the world should have equal access to the practice and benefits of science. Dr. Saha focuses on pediatric preventable infectious diseases, with the goals of (1) using state-of-the-art technology like on-site metagenomics to identify etiologies that elude standard laboratory testing in low- and middle-income countries, and (2) understanding the indirect impacts of interventions like vaccines on the overall health system. She advocates for equal access to scholarly literature and science education. As a team, their mission is to break free of the vicious cycle of limited resources that leads to lack of data required for evidence-based policy decisions, which leads back to limited resources; instead the team is committed to building virtuous cycles of data generation that are sustainable and cost-effective.

Ranga Sampath, Ph.D., joined the Foundation for Innovative New Diagnostics (FIND) as its Chief Scientific Officer in September 2017, where he leads the organization's research and development (R&D) and clinical departments, and will contribute to shaping and implementing FIND's portfolio strategies. Dr. Sampath is a key member of FIND's Executive Management team, which defines the overall business strategy and direction of the organization, mobilizing resources to enable the implementation of FIND's mission. Prior to this, Dr. Sampath served as a Volwiler Senior Research Fellow and the Senior Director of R&D for the Ibis Division of Abbott. He led Ibis's R&D efforts in infectious disease diagnostics, antimicrobial resistance (AMR) diagnostics and surveillance, and was responsible for applications development, validation, data analysis, and reporting for the Ibis polymerase chain reaction/electrospray ionization mass spectrometry–based IRIDICA platform. Dr. Sampath was the cofounder of Ibis Biosciences, Inc., and a co-inventor of the IRIDICA (conformite Europeenne in vitro diagnostic medical) infectious disease diagnostics platform. Dr. Sampath is a recognized leader in the field, with more than 200 publications and presentations and more than 40 issued patents in infectious disease diagnostics. He was an invited participant at the White House National Forum on Antibiotic Stewardship and was an active member of the AdvamedDx Industry Forum for the global commitment on developing diagnostic tests to fight AMR. He has been an invited speaker at many public forums such as the Institute of Medicine, Infectious Diseases Society of America (IDSA), and Parenteral Drug Association (PDA). He was a key member of a U.S. Food and Drug Administration/PDA task force involved in defining the future of viral screening for cell substrates. Dr. Sampath is currently serving his first of a 3-year term as a member of the Diagnostics Committee for IDSA. His research interests include antimicrobial strategy development, pathogen discovery, fevers of unknown origin, tropical diseases, epidemiological surveillance, and biothreat detection.

Peter Sands, M.P.A., became the Executive Director of The Global Fund to Fight AIDS, Tuberculosis and Malaria in March 2018. Mr. Sands is the former Chief Executive Officer (CEO) of Standard Chartered PLC, one of the world's leading international banks operating across more than 70 markets, primarily in emerging markets. After a distinguished career in banking, Mr. Sands was a research fellow at the Harvard Global Health Institute and the Mossavar-Rahmani Center for Business and Government at the Harvard Kennedy School, where he immersed himself in a range of global public health projects. In 2016–2017, Mr. Sands chaired the International Working Group on Financing Pandemic Preparedness at the World Bank. In 2015–2016, he was Chair of the U.S. National Academy of Medicine's Commission on a Global Health Risk Framework for the Future, which published the influential report *The Neglected Dimension of Global Security: A Framework to Counter Infectious Disease Threats* in January 2016. Mr. Sands is also a member of the U.S. National Academies of Sciences, Engineering, and Medicine's Forum on Microbial Threats and is serving on a Committee on Ensuring Access to Affordable Drugs. Mr. Sands served as the CEO of Standard Chartered PLC from 2006 to 2015, having joined the bank in 2002 as the Group Finance Director. Under his leadership, Standard Chartered successfully navigated the turbulence of the global financial crisis in 2007–2009, continuing to support clients and counterparties throughout the worst of the financial stresses and without drawing on government support of any kind. Mr. Sands led Standard Chartered's transformation into one of the world's leading international banks, reinforcing its focus on emerging markets and driving the development of world-class product, risk management, and technology capabilities, underpinned by a highly collaborative culture. During Mr. Sands's tenure as the CEO, Standard Chartered focused its corporate responsibility initiatives on health issues, including avoidable blindness, AIDS, and malaria. Mr. Sands served on the board of the Global Business Coalition on AIDS, Tuberculosis, and Malaria and was the Lead Non-Executive Director on the board of the United Kingdom's Department of Health. After stepping down from the bank in 2015, Mr. Sands has deployed his skills and experience in international finance in global health. Mr. Sands has chaired and participated in a range of high-profile initiatives and has published articles on global health and epidemics in various peer-reviewed journals. His published works on global health include "The Neglected Dimension of Global Security—A Framework for Countering Infectious-Disease Crises," in the *New England Journal of Medicine*, January 2016; "A Stitch in Time Saves Nine: Financing Pandemic Preparedness Through Domestic Resource Mobilization," *Global Health & Diplomacy*, April 2016; "Assessing Economic Vulnerability to Infectious Disease Outbreaks," *The Lancet*, May 2016; "Beyond the Ebola Battle—Winning the War Against Future Epidemics," *British Medical Journal*, January 2017; and "From Panic and Neglect to Investing in Health Security: Financing Pandemic Preparedness at a National Level," *World Bank*, May 2017. Mr. Sands has served on numerous boards and commissions, including as a governor of the United Kingdom's National Institute for Economic and Social Research, as a member of the International Advisory Board of the Monetary Authority of Singapore, as the Board Director of the Institute of International Finance, and as a Director of the World Economic Forum. Born in the United Kingdom, the son of a naval officer and an artist, Mr. Sands was educated in Canada, Malaysia, the United Kingdom, and the United States. He began his career in the United Kingdom's Foreign Office and then joined McKinsey & Company, where he worked for 13 years in the London office, advising clients in the financial services and telecommunications sectors. Mr. Sands graduated from Brasenose College, Oxford University, with a First Class degree in politics, philosophy, and economics. He also received an M.P.A. from Harvard University, where he was a Harkness Fellow.

Carrie Teicher, M.D., M.P.H., is the Director of Programs at Doctors Without Borders/Médecins Sans Frontières (MSF). The Programs Department supports multiple dossiers including but not limited to work on advocacy, global health diplomacy, research, and innovation. Prior to this role, she worked for 7 years as a medical and surgical epidemiologist with Epicentre (www.epicentre.msf.org), MSF's internal research and epidemiological institute. Dr. Teicher has worked with MSF in multiple different roles and numerous contexts throughout four continents. Outside of MSF, Dr. Teicher has additionally served as a medical coordinator, primary investigator, or program coordinator in the global health sector working primarily in the emergency medicine and tropical medicine fields. She holds an M.D. from the Sackler School of Medicine, an M.P.H. from the Mailman School of Public Health at Columbia University, and an undergraduate degree from Barnard College. From 2001 to 2003 she served in the Peace Corps in Mali.

Jonathan Towner, Ph.D., works in the Viral Special Pathogens Branch at the U.S. Centers for Disease Control and Prevention (CDC). His team focuses primarily on ecological aspects of Ebola and Marburg virus biology with emphasis on identifying their reservoir hosts. Dr. Towner's team also studies the mechanisms used by these viruses to persist in nature long term, and potential drivers of virus spillover to humans. Recent accomplishments include the discovery of the Egyptian fruit bat (*Rousettus aegyptiacus*), the only known filovirus reservoir, as a natural reservoir for Marburg virus, and the discovery of Bundibugyo ebolavirus, the newest member of the *Ebolavirus* genus. In addition to his ecological investigations, Dr. Towner responds on occasion to filovirus outbreaks in Africa to operate molecular diagnostic field labs. In this capacity, he has established or operated diagnostic labs at four major filovirus outbreaks since 2000, including the CDC lab in Bo, Sierra Leone, in October 2014. Dr. Towner has been well trained in filovirus biology and ecology by leading authorities in the field, including Drs. Stuart Nichol, Thomas Ksiazek, Robert Swanepoel, and Pierre Rollin. Dr. Towner has more than 22 years of training as a molecular virologist and 17 years of experience conducting virus research under biosafety level-4 containment.

Maurizio Vecchione is the Executive Vice President of Global Good and Research at Intellectual Ventures (IV). In this role, Mr. Vecchione oversees Global Good, IV's collaboration with Bill Gates to invent and deploy technology specifically focused on improving life in developing countries, as well as the research and operations of the Intellectual Ventures Laboratory (IV Lab) and Institute for Disease Modeling. Under his leadership, Global Good and IV Lab engage in cutting-edge research and invention for the benefit of humanity around global health and global development priorities. He has nearly 30 years of experience in research and the technology sector, most recently serving as the Chief Executive Officer (CEO) of Arrogene and prior to that as the CEO of telemedicine pioneer CompuMed. He has contributed to building 9 start-ups and helped launch more than 50 commercial products, resulting in more than $1 billion in shareholder value. His work spans the software, Internet, wireless, and life sciences sectors, primarily in connection with translational sciences for science derived from government and academic research and development efforts. Mr. Vecchione is involved in several nonprofit initiatives, including his role as cofounder and member of the board of ReefQuest, a global organization focused on fostering marine environmental stewardship in children through citizen science. An inventor, he is named on multiple U.S. patents and patent applications related to imaging, image processing, and nano-bio-polymer and telecommunications technologies. Mr. Vecchione studied physics at the University of California, Berkeley.

Rajeev Venkayya, M.D., is the President of Takeda's Global Vaccine Business Unit, a vertically integrated business with a pipeline that includes vaccine candidates for norovirus and dengue. He also oversees Takeda's contract with the U.S. Biomedical Advanced Research and Development Authority to develop a vaccine to support the Zika response in the United States and affected regions around the world. He is an independent member of the board of CEPI, the Coalition for Epidemic Preparedness Innovations, and a life member of the Council on Foreign Relations. Prior to Takeda, Dr. Venkayya served as the Director of Vaccine Delivery in the Global Health Program at the Bill & Melinda Gates Foundation, where he was responsible for the Gates Foundation's efforts in polio eradication and new vaccine introduction, and a grant portfolio of $500 million per year. While at the Gates Foundation, he served on the Board of the Global Alliance for Vaccines and Immunization. Dr. Venkayya was previously the Special Assistant to the President for Biodefense at the White House. In this capacity, he oversaw U.S. preparedness for bioterrorism and biological threats and was responsible for the development and implementation of the National Strategy for Pandemic Influenza. He first came to Washington, DC, through the nonpartisan White House Fellowship program in 2002. Trained in pulmonary and critical care medicine, Dr. Venkayya served as an Assistant Professor of Medicine in the Division of Pulmonary and Critical Care Medicine at the University of California, San Francisco. He also served as Co-Director of the Medical Intensive Care Unit and the Director of the High-Risk Asthma Clinic at San Francisco General Hospital. Dr. Venkayya was a resident and the Chief Medical Resident in internal medicine at the University of Michigan. He completed his undergraduate and medical school education in the B.S./M.D. program at the Northeast Ohio Universities College of Medicine in the United States, where he was inducted into the Alpha Omega Alpha honorary medical society.

Sabrina Welsh, M.P.H., brings more than 10 years of international clinical trial and program management experience to her role at the Human Vaccines Project. As the Director of Programs and Operations, Ms. Welsh oversees the clinical and lab operations within the Project's network to help the Project run efficiently to produce high-quality and impactful data. Before joining the Human Vaccines Project, Ms. Welsh worked as the Senior Clinical Program Manager for the International AIDS Vaccine Initiative (IAVI), where she led early clinical development project teams for vaccines and monoclonal antibodies for the prevention of HIV and other emerging infectious diseases. She also helped develop the program for Epidemiology for Vaccine Advancement, Capacity and Science (EpiVACS) at IAVI, where her work focused on acute HIV infection and access to health care in marginalized key populations. She received an M.P.H. from the New York University College of Global Public Health and a B.S. with distinction in research from Cornell University.